Easy Smoothie Recipe for Ramadan

"30 Quick and Nutritious Blends to Energize Your Ramadan Fasts"

Dr. Fathum

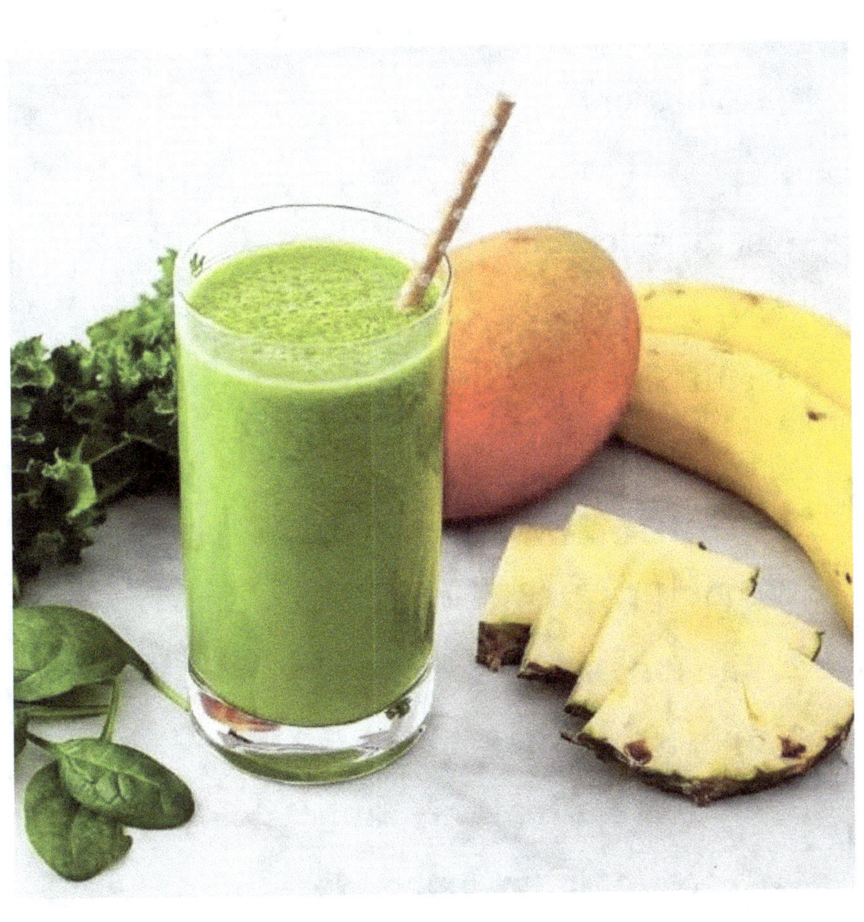

Table of contents

9. Peach Ginger Smoothie

10. Watermelon Basil Smoothie

11. Carrot Orange Smoothie

12. Mango Turmeric Smoothie

13. Raspberry Beet Smoothie

14. Apple Cinnamon Smoothie

15. Strawberry Kiwi Smoothie

16. Peanut Butter Banana Smoothie

17. Mixed Berry Chia Smoothie

18. Chocolate Almond Smoothie

19. Tropical Green Smoothie

20. Matcha Green Tea Smoothie

21. Pomegranate Berry Smoothie

22. Vanilla Almond Smoothie

23. Chocolate Banana Smoothie

24. Cantaloupe Mint Smoothie

25. Coconut Mango Smoothie

Conclusion.

Introduction

Welcome to "30 Easy Smoothie Recipes for Ramadan: Quick and Nutritious Blends to Energize Your Fasts"! As the holy month of Ramadan approaches, many individuals embark on a journey of spiritual reflection and self-discipline through fasting. Fasting during Ramadan involves abstaining from food and drink from dawn until sunset, making it essential to choose nutrient-rich foods that provide sustained energy and hydration during non-fasting hours.

In this book, we've curated a collection of 30 delicious and easy-to-make smoothie recipes specifically designed to support your Ramadan fasts. These smoothies are crafted with care to provide a balance of essential nutrients, vitamins, and minerals to help you stay energized, hydrated, and nourished throughout the day.

Whether you're looking for a refreshing drink to break your fast, a nutritious meal to start your day, or a satisfying snack to enjoy between meals, you'll find a variety of options to suit your taste preferences and dietary needs. From vibrant fruit combinations to creamy nutty blends, each recipe is thoughtfully crafted to provide both flavor and nutritional benefits.

Join us on a journey to revitalize your Ramadan fasts with these quick and nutritious smoothie recipes. Here's to a month filled with hea, and spiritual growth.

What Is Smoothie

A smoothie is a thick, creamy beverage made by blending together a combination of fruits, vegetables, liquids (such as water, milk, juice, or yogurt), and sometimes ice or other ingredients like protein powder, nuts, seeds, or sweeteners. The ingredients are blended until smooth, resulting in a drinkable mixture that can be enjoyed as a snack, meal replacement, or refreshing treat.

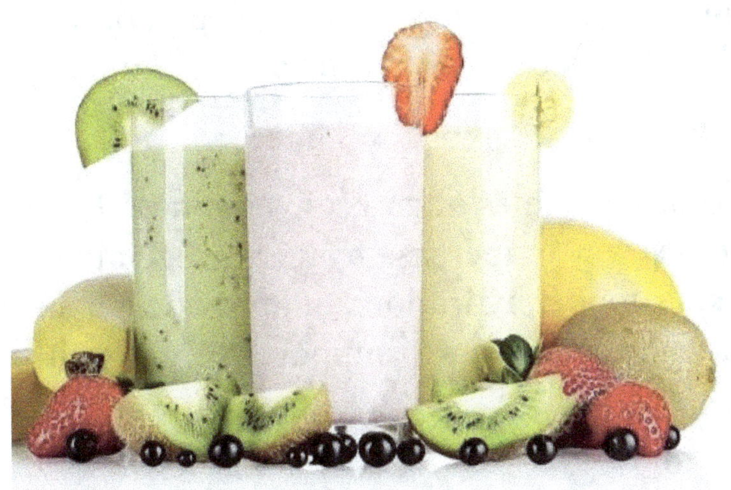

Smoothies are highly customizable, allowing individuals to tailor them to their taste preferences and nutritional needs. They can range from simple fruit-based blends to more complex combinations incorporating vegetables, protein sources, and superfoods.

Smoothies are popular for their convenience, versatility, and ability to pack a variety of nutrients into one convenient serving. They are often enjoyed as a quick and easy breakfast option, a post-workout recovery drink, or a healthy snack throughout the day.

Overall, smoothies offer a convenient and delicious way to increase fruit and vegetable intake, support hydration, and provide a boost of energy and nutrients to support overall health and well-being.

Health benefits of smoothies

Smoothies offer a variety of health benefits, making them a popular choice for those seeking a convenient and nutritious way to consume a variety of fruits, vegetables, and other wholesome ingredients. Here are some of the key health benefits of incorporating smoothies into your diet:

1. Nutrient-Rich: Smoothies provide a convenient way to pack a variety of nutrients into one delicious drink. Fruits, vegetables, nuts, seeds, and other ingredients used in smoothies are rich in vitamins, minerals, antioxidants, and fiber, which are essential for overall health and well-being.

2. Hydration: Many smoothie recipes include hydrating ingredients such as fruits, vegetables, and liquids like water, coconut water, or milk. Consuming smoothies can help keep you hydrated, especially

important during hot weather or periods of increased physical activity.

3. Digestive Health: Smoothies can support digestive health due to their high fiber content from ingredients like fruits, vegetables, and seeds. Fiber helps promote regular bowel movements, prevent constipation, and support a healthy gut microbiome.

4. Weight Management: Incorporating smoothies into a balanced diet can aid in weight management. They provide a satisfying and filling option that can help control appetite and reduce the likelihood of overeating. Additionally, smoothies can be tailored to include ingredients that support metabolism and fat burning.

5. Energy Boost: The natural sugars found in fruits provide a quick source of energy, making smoothies an excellent choice for a pre-workout snack or a morning pick-me-up. Adding ingredients like nuts, seeds, or protein powder can further enhance the energy-boosting effects of smoothies.

6. Immune Support: Smoothies made with ingredients rich in vitamin C, antioxidants, and other immune-boosting nutrients can help support a healthy immune system. Regular consumption of these nutrient-dense beverages may help reduce the risk of infections and illnesses.

7. Convenience: Smoothies are quick and easy to prepare, making them a convenient option for busy individuals or those with hectic lifestyles. They can be enjoyed on-

the-go as a meal replacement, snack, or post-workout recovery drink.

8. Versatility: The versatility of smoothies allows for endless flavor combinations and ingredient variations. Whether you prefer fruity, green, creamy, or indulgent flavors, there's a smoothie recipe to suit every taste preference and dietary requirement.

In summary, smoothies offer a delicious and convenient way to boost your intake of essential nutrients, support overall health, and promote hydration and digestive wellness. Incorporating smoothies into your diet can be a simple yet effective way to nourish your body and enhance your well-being.

30 Smoothie Recipes, Ingredients, duration, preparation.

1. Banana Date Smoothie

Ingredients:

- 1 ripe banana

- 3-4 dates, pitted

- 1 cup milk (dairy or plant-based)

- Pinch of cinnamon (optional)

Minutes for Preparation: 5 minutes

How to Prepare:

1. Peel the banana and break it into chunks.

2. Remove the pits from the dates if they're not already pitted.

3. In a blender, combine the banana chunks, pitted dates, milk, and a pinch of cinnamon if desired.

4. Blend until smooth and creamy.

5. Pour into glasses and serve immediately.

Health Benefits in Ramadan:

- Energy Boost: Bananas are rich in carbohydrates, providing a quick energy boost during fasting hours.

- Hydration: The high water content in bananas helps in maintaining hydration levels during fasting.

- Digestive Health: Dates are rich in fiber, which aids digestion and helps prevent constipation, which can be common during Ramadan.

- Nutrient-Rich: Dates are also packed with essential nutrients like potassium, magnesium, and vitamins, which are beneficial for overall health and well-being during fasting.

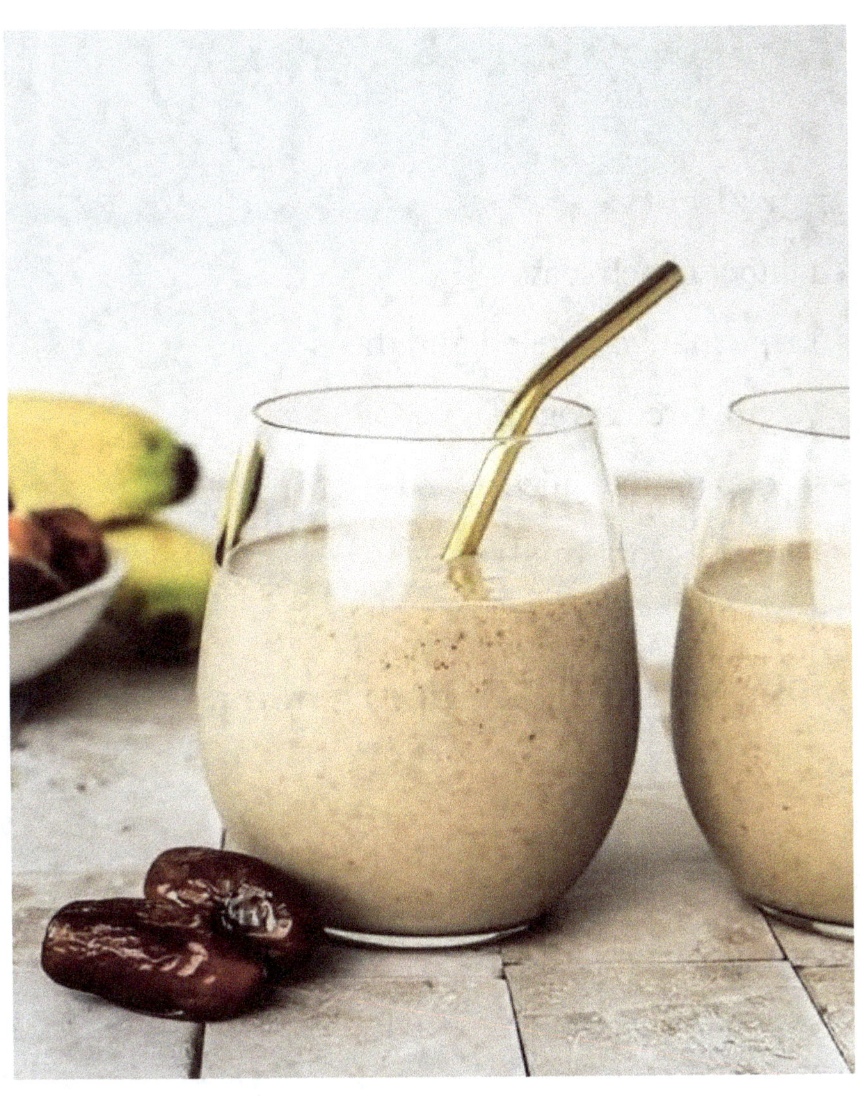

2.Spinach Mango Smoothie

Ingredients:

- 1 cup spinach leaves

- 1 ripe mango, peeled and diced

- ½ cup Greek yogurt

- ½ cup orange juice

- Ice cubes (optional)

Minutes for Preparation: 5 minutes

How to Prepare:

1. Wash the spinach leaves thoroughly and place them in a blender.

2. Add the diced mango to the blender.

3. Spoon in the Greek yogurt and pour in the orange juice.

4. If desired, add a few ice cubes to the blender to make the smoothie colder.

5. Blend all the ingredients until smooth and creamy.

6. Pour the smoothie into glasses and serve immediately.

Health Benefits in Ramadan:

- Hydration: Mangoes have high water content, which helps in keeping the body hydrated during fasting hours.

- Vitamins and Minerals: Spinach is rich in vitamins A, C, and K, as well as iron and folate, providing essential nutrients during Ramadan.

- Digestive Health: Spinach is also high in fiber, which aids in digestion and helps maintain digestive health during fasting.

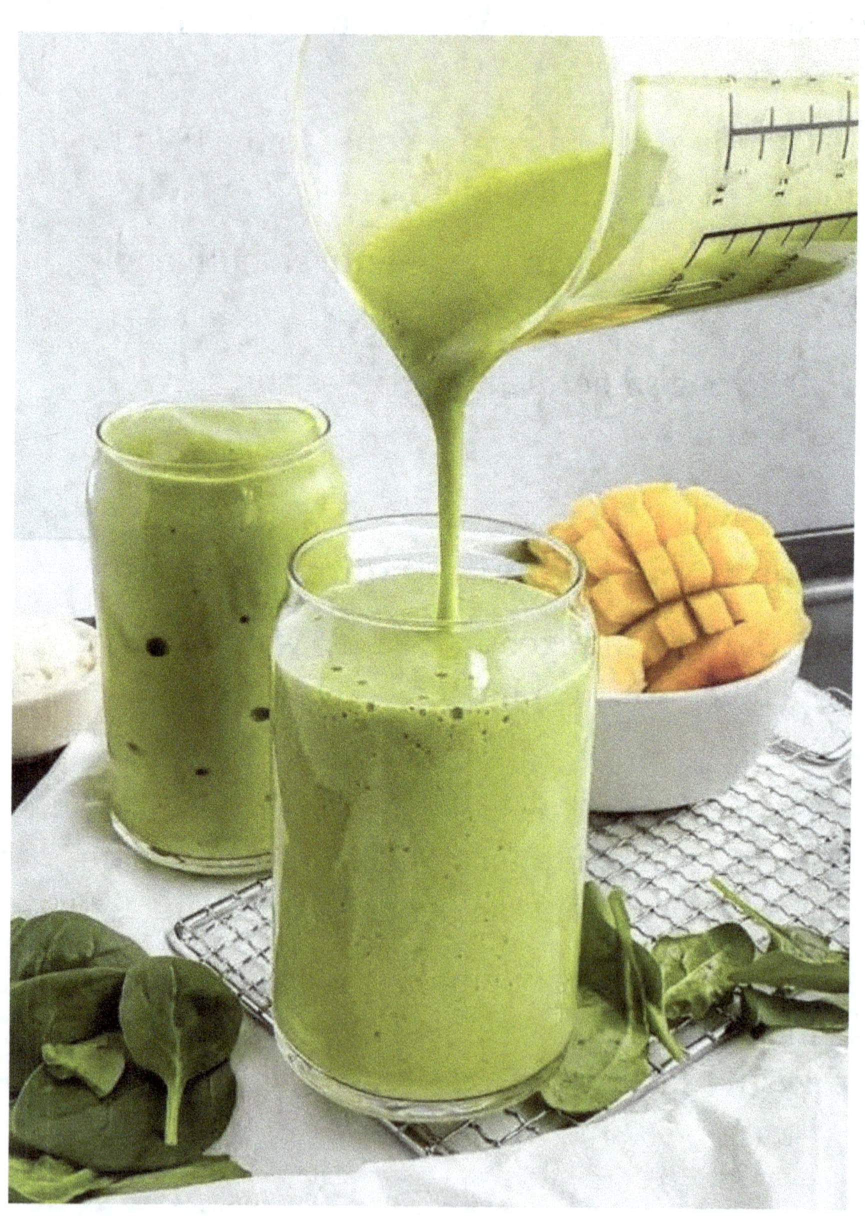

3.Almond Butter Berry Smoothie

Here's the recipe for the Almond Butter Berry Smoothie:

Ingredients:

- 1 cup mixed berries (such as strawberries, blueberries, raspberries)

- 1 tablespoon almond butter

- ½ cup almond milk (or any milk of your choice)

- ½ cup Greek yogurt

- Honey or maple syrup to taste (optional)

Minutes for Preparation: 5 minutes

How to Prepare:

1. Wash the mixed berries and add them to a blender.

2. Spoon in the almond butter.

3. Pour in the almond milk and add the Greek yogurt.

4. Optionally, add honey or maple syrup for sweetness.

5. Blend all the ingredients until smooth and creamy.

6. Taste and adjust sweetness if needed by adding more honey or maple syrup.

7. Pour the smoothie into glasses and serve immediately.

Health Benefits in Ramadan:

- Protein and Healthy Fats: Almond butter provides protein and healthy fats, which help keep you feeling full and satisfied during the fasting period.

- Antioxidants: Berries are rich in antioxidants, which help fight inflammation and oxidative stress in the body, supporting overall health during Ramadan.

- Nutrient-Rich: Greek yogurt adds calcium and probiotics, which are beneficial for bone health and gut health, respectively, during fasting.

- Energy Boost: The combination of protein, healthy fats, and carbohydrates from the berries provides sustained energy throughout the day.

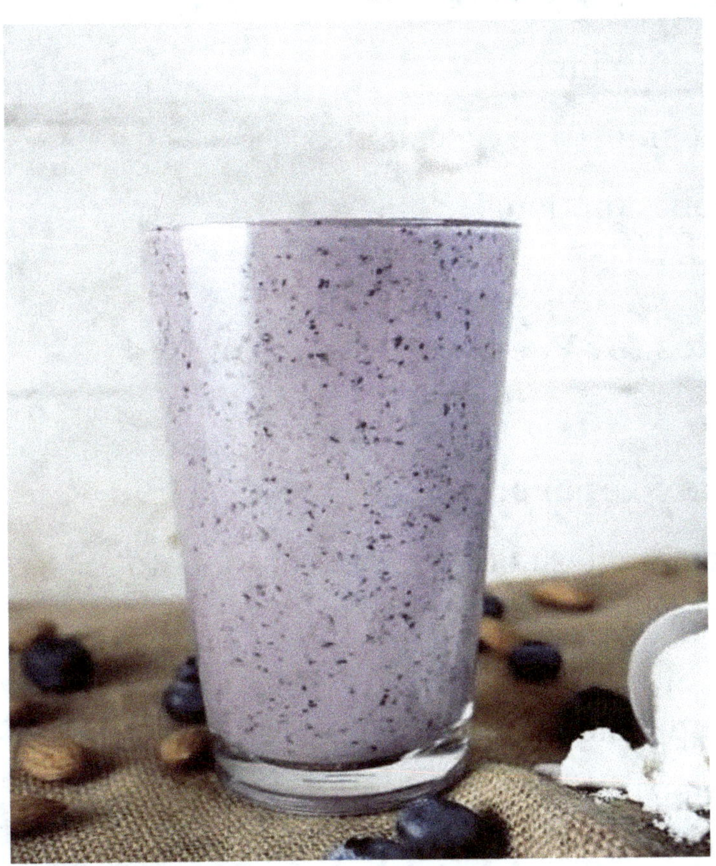

4. Avocado Honey smoothie

Ingredients:

- 1 ripe avocado, peeled and pitted

- 1 tablespoon honey

- ½ cup Greek yogurt

- Juice of ½ lime

- ½ cup milk (dairy or plant-based)

- Ice cubes (optional)

Minutes for Preparation: 5 minutes

How to Prepare:

1. Scoop the flesh of the ripe avocado into a blender.

2. Add the honey, Greek yogurt, lime juice, and milk to the blender.

3. Optionally, add a few ice cubes for a colder smoothie.

4. Blend all the ingredients until smooth and creamy.

5. Taste the smoothie and adjust sweetness or tanginess by adding more honey or lime juice if desired.

6. Pour the smoothie into glasses and serve immediately.

Health Benefits in Ramadan:

- Healthy Fats: Avocado provides healthy monounsaturated fats, which help keep you feeling full and satisfied during fasting.

- Hydration: Avocado contains a high water content, contributing to hydration during the fasting period.

- Vitamins and Minerals: Avocado is rich in vitamins and minerals, including potassium, vitamin K, vitamin E, and folate, providing essential nutrients during Ramadan.

- Digestive Health: The fiber in avocado helps promote digestive health and prevent constipation, which can be beneficial during fasting.

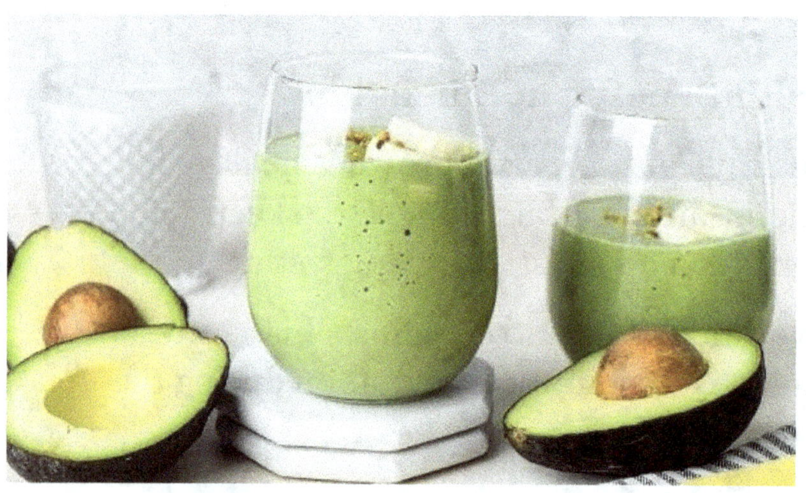

5. Pineapple Coconut Smoothie

Ingredients:

- 1 cup chopped pineapple

- ½ cup coconut milk

- ½ banana

- ¼ cup Greek yogurt

- Ice cubes (optional)

Minutes for Preparation: 5 minutes

How to Prepare:

1. Place the chopped pineapple, coconut milk, banana, and Greek yogurt in a blender.

2. Optionally, add some ice cubes for a colder smoothie.

3. Blend all the ingredients until smooth and creamy.

4. Taste the smoothie and adjust sweetness by adding more banana if desired.

5. Blend again until well incorporated.

6. Pour the smoothie into glasses and serve immediately.

Health Benefits in Ramadan:

- Hydration: Pineapple and coconut milk both have high water content, contributing to hydration during fasting.

- Vitamins and Minerals: Pineapple is rich in vitamin C, manganese, and antioxidants, while coconut milk provides essential nutrients like potassium and magnesium, supporting overall health during Ramadan.

- Digestive Health: The fiber in pineapple helps promote digestive health and regular bowel movements, which can be beneficial during fasting.

- Energy Boost: The natural sugars in pineapple and banana provide a quick energy boost during fasting hours.

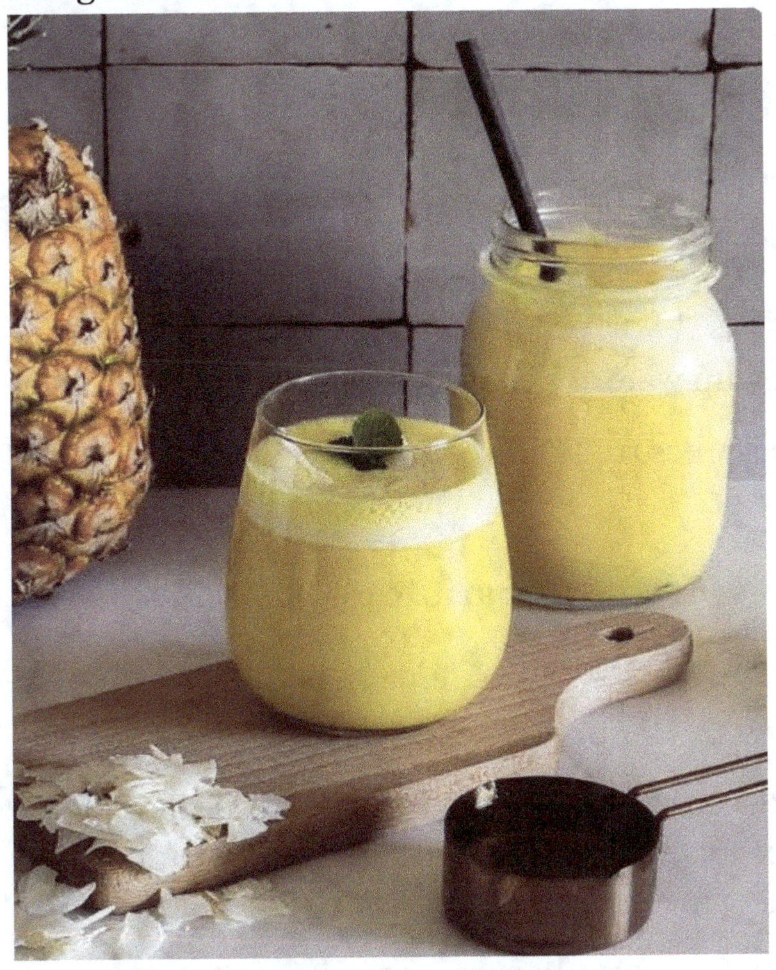

6. Cucumber Mint Smoothie

Ingredients:

- 1 cucumber, peeled and chopped

- Handful of fresh mint leaves

- ½ cup Greek yogurt

- Juice of ½ lemon

- ½ cup water or coconut water

- Ice cubes (optional)

Minutes for Preparation: 5 minutes

How to Prepare:

1. Place the chopped cucumber, fresh mint leaves, Greek yogurt, lemon juice, and water (or coconut water) in a blender.

2. Optionally, add some ice cubes for a colder smoothie.

3. Blend all the ingredients until smooth and well combined.

4. Taste the smoothie and adjust the flavor by adding more lemon juice or mint leaves if desired.

5. Blend again until the desired consistency is reached.

6. Pour the smoothie into glasses and serve immediately.

Health Benefits in Ramadan:

- Hydration: Cucumber and coconut water have high water content, aiding in hydration during fasting.

- Digestive Health: Cucumber is hydrating and contains fiber, promoting digestive health and preventing constipation during Ramadan.

- Refreshing: The combination of cucumber and mint provides a refreshing flavor, helping to combat thirst and refresh the palate during fasting hours.

- Vitamins and Minerals: Mint is rich in vitamins A and C, while cucumber provides essential nutrients like potassium and magnesium, supporting overall health during Ramadan.

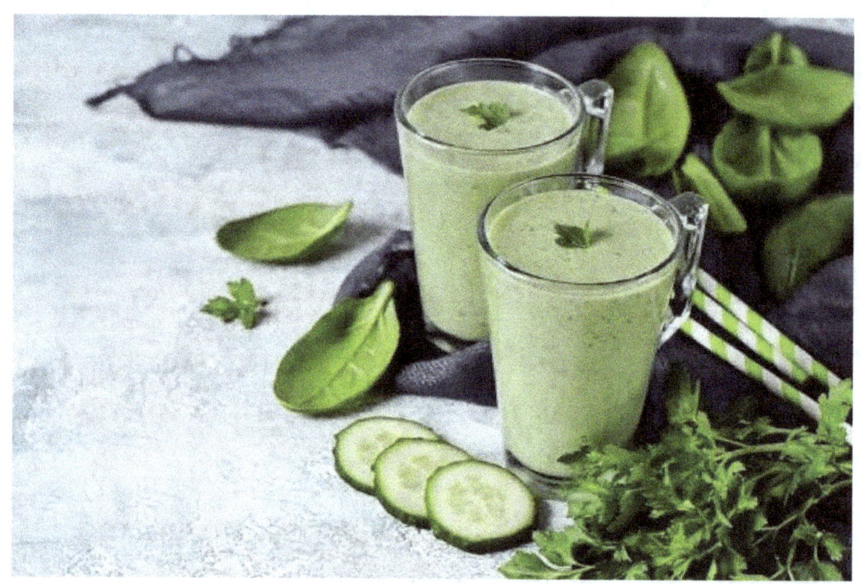

7. Cherry Almond Smoothie

Ingredients:

- 1 cup pitted cherries

- 1 tablespoon almond butter

- ½ cup almond milk (or any milk of your choice)

- ½ cup Greek yogurt

- Honey or maple syrup to taste (optional)

- Ice cubes (optional)

Minutes for Preparation: 5 minutes

How to Prepare:

1. Wash the pitted cherries and place them in a blender.

2. Add the almond butter, almond milk, and Greek yogurt to the blender.

3. Optionally, add honey or maple syrup for sweetness.

4. If desired, add some ice cubes for a colder smoothie.

5. Blend all the ingredients until smooth and creamy.

6. Taste the smoothie and adjust sweetness if needed by adding more honey or maple syrup.

7. Blend again until well combined.

8. Pour the smoothie into glasses and serve immediately.

Health Benefits in Ramadan:

- Antioxidants: Cherries are rich in antioxidants, which help fight inflammation and oxidative stress in the body, supporting overall health during Ramadan.

- Protein and Healthy Fats: Almond butter provides protein and healthy fats, helping to keep you feeling full and satisfied during fasting.

- Nutrient-Rich: Greek yogurt adds calcium and probiotics, beneficial for bone health and gut health, respectively, during fasting.

- Energy Boost: The combination of carbohydrates, protein, and healthy fats in this smoothie provides sustained energy throughout the day.

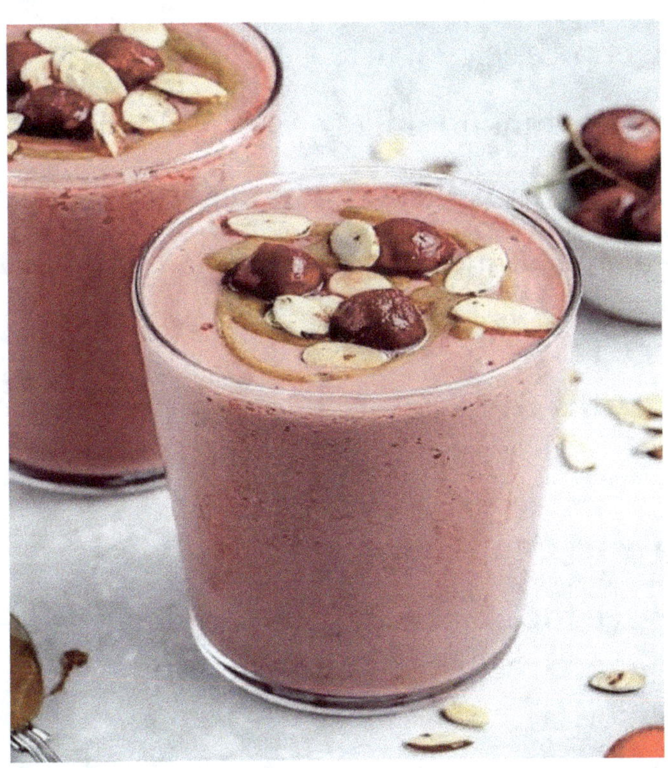

8.Blueberry Kale Smoothie

Ingredients:

- 1 cup fresh or frozen blueberries

- 1 cup chopped kale leaves, stems removed

- ½ banana

- ½ cup Greek yogurt

- ½ cup almond milk (or any milk of your choice)

- Honey or maple syrup to taste (optional)

- Ice cubes (optional)

Minutes for Preparation: 5 minutes

How to Prepare:

1. Place the blueberries, chopped kale leaves, banana, Greek yogurt, and almond milk in a blender.

2. Optionally, add honey or maple syrup for sweetness.

3. If desired, add some ice cubes for a colder smoothie.

4. Blend all the ingredients until smooth and creamy.

5. Taste the smoothie and adjust sweetness if needed by adding more honey or maple syrup.

6. Blend again until well combined.

7. Pour the smoothie into glasses and serve immediately.

Health Benefits in Ramadan:

- Nutrient-Rich: Blueberries are packed with antioxidants, vitamins, and minerals, providing essential nutrients during fasting.

- Hydration: Both blueberries and kale have high water content, contributing to hydration during fasting.

- Digestive Health: Kale is rich in fiber, promoting digestive health and regular bowel movements, which can be beneficial during Ramadan.

- Energy Boost: The natural sugars in blueberries and banana provide a quick energy boost during fasting hours.

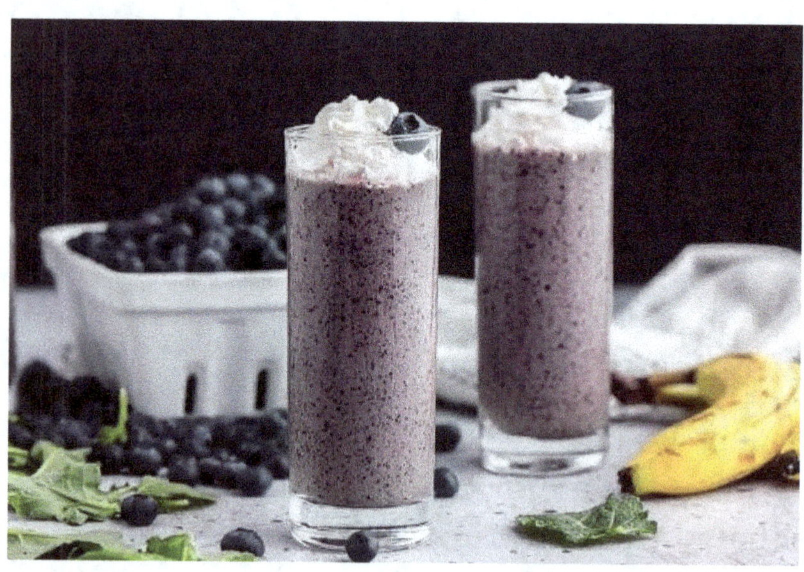

9.Peach Ginger Smoothie

Ingredients:

- 1 ripe peach, pitted and sliced

- 1 teaspoon grated ginger

- ½ cup Greek yogurt

- ½ cup orange juice

- Honey or maple syrup to taste (optional)

- Ice cubes (optional)

Minutes for Preparation: 5 minutes

How to Prepare:

1. Place the sliced peach, grated ginger, Greek yogurt, and orange juice in a blender.

2. Optionally, add honey or maple syrup for sweetness.

3. If desired, add some ice cubes for a colder smoothie.

4. Blend all the ingredients until smooth and creamy.

5. Taste the smoothie and adjust sweetness if needed by adding more honey or maple syrup.

6. Blend again until well combined.

7. Pour the smoothie into glasses and serve immediately.

Health Benefits in Ramadan:

- Digestive Health: Ginger helps soothe the stomach and aids digestion, which can be beneficial during Ramadan, especially after breaking the fast.

- Vitamin C: Peaches and orange juice are rich in vitamin C, which supports the immune system, helping to prevent illness during Ramadan.

- Hydration: Both peaches and orange juice have high water content, contributing to hydration during fasting.

- Antioxidants: Peaches contain antioxidants like vitamin A and vitamin C, which help fight inflammation and support overall health during Ramadan.

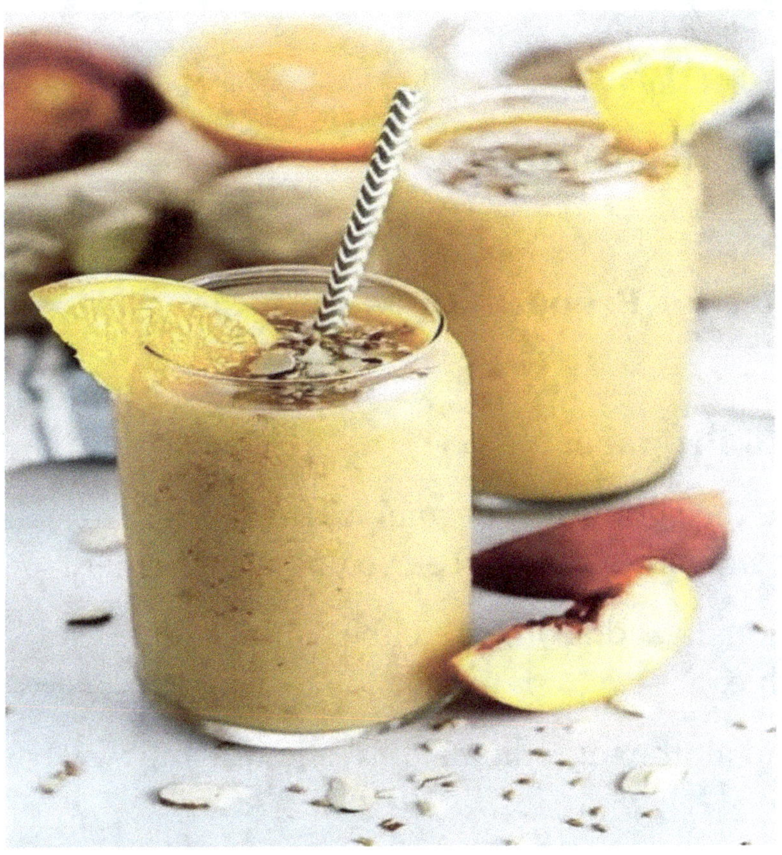

10. Watermelon Basil Smoothie

Ingredients:

- 2 cups chopped watermelon, seeds removed

- Handful of fresh basil leaves

- Juice of ½ lime

- ½ cup Greek yogurt

- Ice cubes (optional)

Minutes for Preparation: 5 minutes

How to Prepare:

1. Place the chopped watermelon, fresh basil leaves, lime juice, and Greek yogurt in a blender.

2. Optionally, add some ice cubes for a colder smoothie.

3. Blend all the ingredients until smooth and well combined.

4. Taste the smoothie and adjust the flavor by adding more lime juice or basil leaves if desired.

5. Blend again until the desired consistency is reached.

6. Pour the smoothie into glasses and serve immediately.

Health Benefits in Ramadan:

- Hydration: Watermelon has high water content, contributing to hydration during fasting.

- Vitamins and Minerals: Watermelon is rich in vitamins A and C, as well as potassium, providing essential nutrients during Ramadan.

- Digestive Health: Basil helps soothe the stomach and aids digestion, which can be beneficial during Ramadan, especially after breaking the fast.

- Refreshing: The combination of watermelon and basil provides a refreshing flavor, helping to combat thirst and refresh the palate during fasting

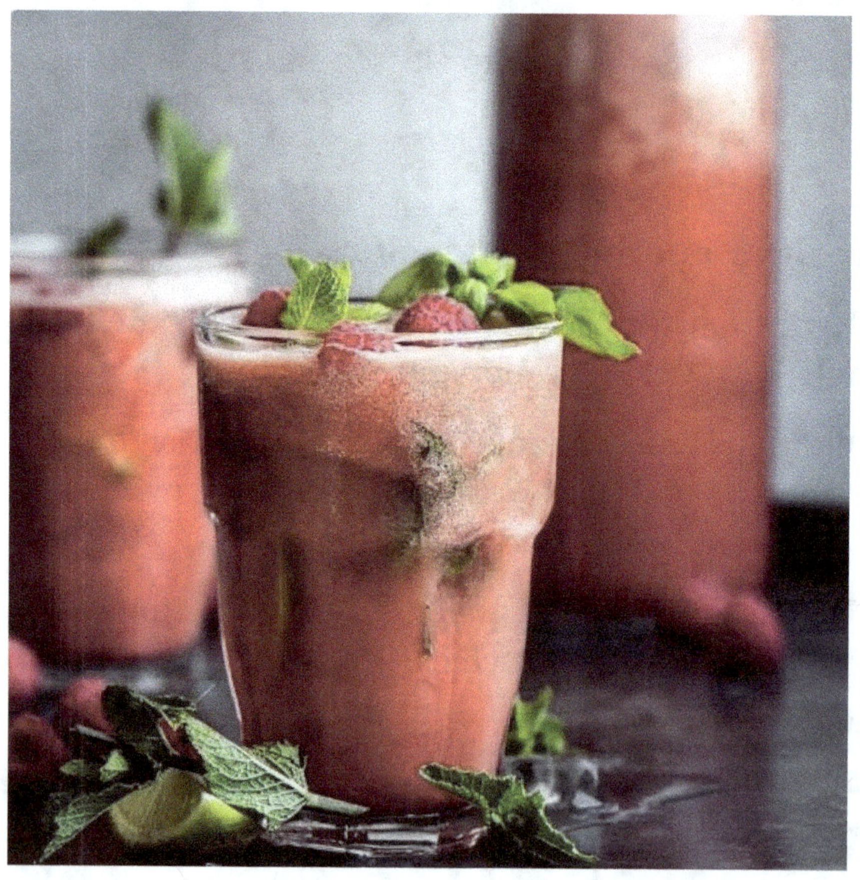

11. Carrot Orange Smoothie

Ingredients:

- 1 large carrot, peeled and chopped

- Juice of 2 oranges

- ½ cup Greek yogurt

- ½ teaspoon ground turmeric

- Honey or maple syrup to taste (optional)

- Ice cubes (optional)

Minutes for Preparation: 5 minutes

How to Prepare:

1. Place the chopped carrot, orange juice, Greek yogurt, and ground turmeric in a blender.

2. Optionally, add honey or maple syrup for sweetness.

3. If desired, add some ice cubes for a colder smoothie.

4. Blend all the ingredients until smooth and creamy.

5. Taste the smoothie and adjust sweetness if needed by adding more honey or maple syrup.

6. Blend again until well combined.

7. Pour the smoothie into glasses and serve immediately.

Health Benefits in Ramadan:

- Vitamin C: Oranges are rich in vitamin C, which supports the immune system, helping to prevent illness during Ramadan.

- Digestive Health: Carrots are high in fiber, promoting digestive health and regular bowel movements, which can be beneficial during Ramadan.

- Anti-Inflammatory: Turmeric has anti-inflammatory properties, which may help reduce inflammation in the body, supporting overall health during Ramadan.

- Hydration: Oranges have high water content, contributing to hydration during fasting.

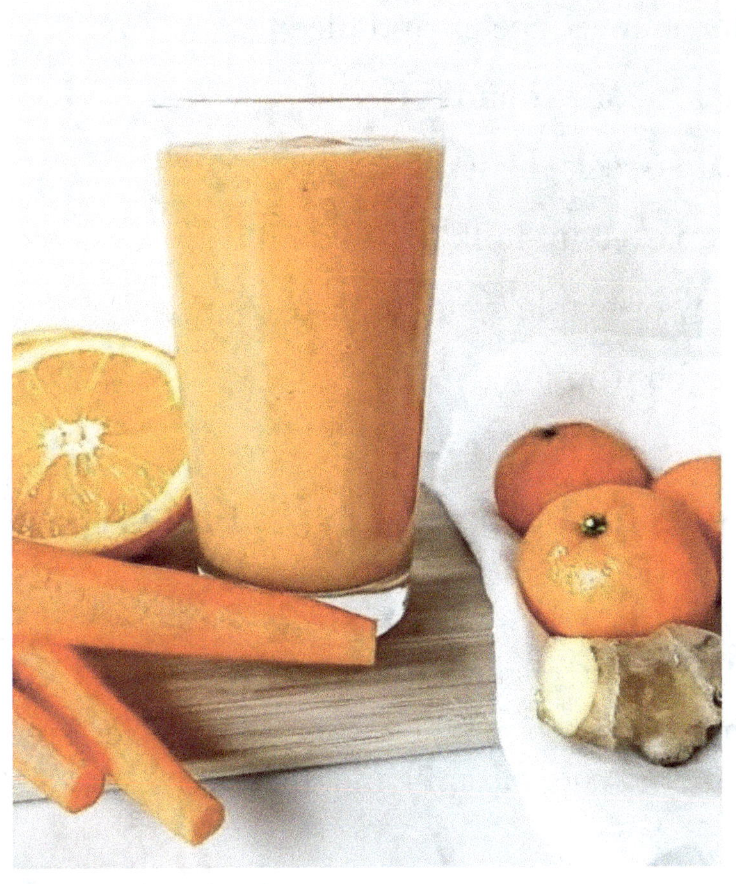

12. Mango Turmeric Smoothie

Ingredients:

- 1 ripe mango, peeled and diced

- ½ teaspoon ground turmeric

- ½ cup Greek yogurt

- ½ cup coconut milk (or any milk of your choice)

- Honey or maple syrup to taste (optional)

- Ice cubes (optional)

Minutes for Preparation: 5 minutes

How to Prepare:

1. Place the diced mango, ground turmeric, Greek yogurt, and coconut milk in a blender.

2. Optionally, add honey or maple syrup for sweetness.

3. If desired, add some ice cubes for a colder smoothie.

4. Blend all the ingredients until smooth and creamy.

5. Taste the smoothie and adjust sweetness if needed by adding more honey or maple syrup.

6. Blend again until well combined.

7. Pour the smoothie into glasses and serve immediately.

Health Benefits in Ramadan:

- Vitamin C: Mangoes are rich in vitamin C, which supports the immune system, helping to prevent illness during Ramadan.

- Digestive Health: Mangoes contain digestive enzymes that aid digestion and promote regular bowel movements, which can be beneficial during Ramadan.

- Anti-Inflammatory: Turmeric has anti-inflammatory properties, which may help reduce inflammation in the body, supporting overall health during Ramadan.

- Hydration: Both mangoes and coconut milk have high water content, contributing to hydration during fasting.

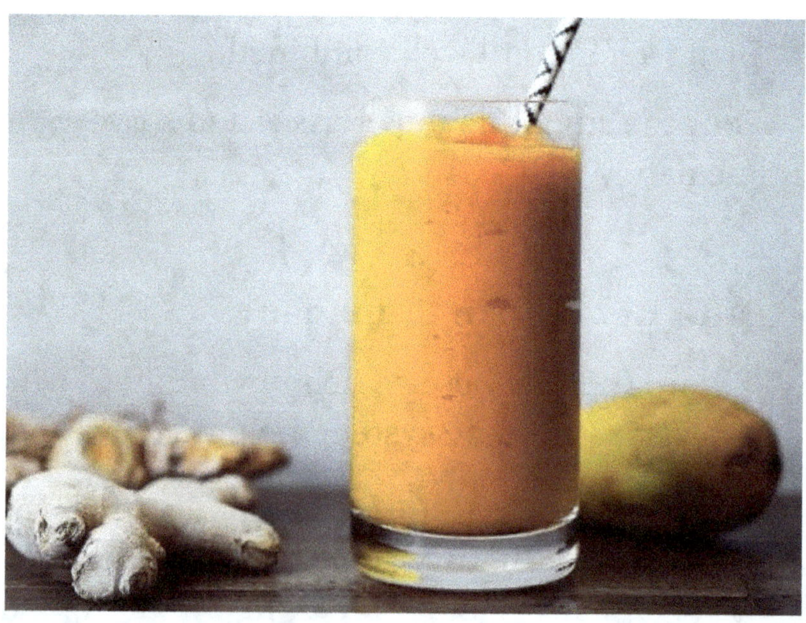

13. Raspberry Beet Smoothie

Ingredients:

- ½ cup raspberries (fresh or frozen)

- 1 small cooked beet, peeled and chopped

- ½ banana

- ½ cup Greek yogurt

- ½ cup almond milk (or any milk of your choice)

- Honey or maple syrup to taste (optional)

- Ice cubes (optional)

Minutes for Preparation: 5 minutes

How to Prepare:

1. Place the raspberries, cooked beet, banana, Greek yogurt, and almond milk in a blender.

2. Optionally, add honey or maple syrup for sweetness.

3. If desired, add some ice cubes for a colder smoothie.

4. Blend all the ingredients until smooth and creamy.

5. Taste the smoothie and adjust sweetness if needed by adding more honey or maple syrup.

6. Blend again until well combined.

7. Pour the smoothie into glasses and serve immediately.

Health Benefits in Ramadan:

- Antioxidants: Raspberries and beets are both rich in antioxidants, which help fight inflammation and oxidative stress in the body, supporting overall health during Ramadan.

- Vitamins and Minerals: Beets are high in folate, manganese, and potassium, while raspberries are packed with vitamin C and fiber, providing essential nutrients during fasting.

- Digestive Health: Both raspberries and beets contain fiber, promoting digestive health and regular bowel movements, which can be beneficial during Ramadan.

- Hydration: Raspberries have high water content, contributing to hydration during fasting.

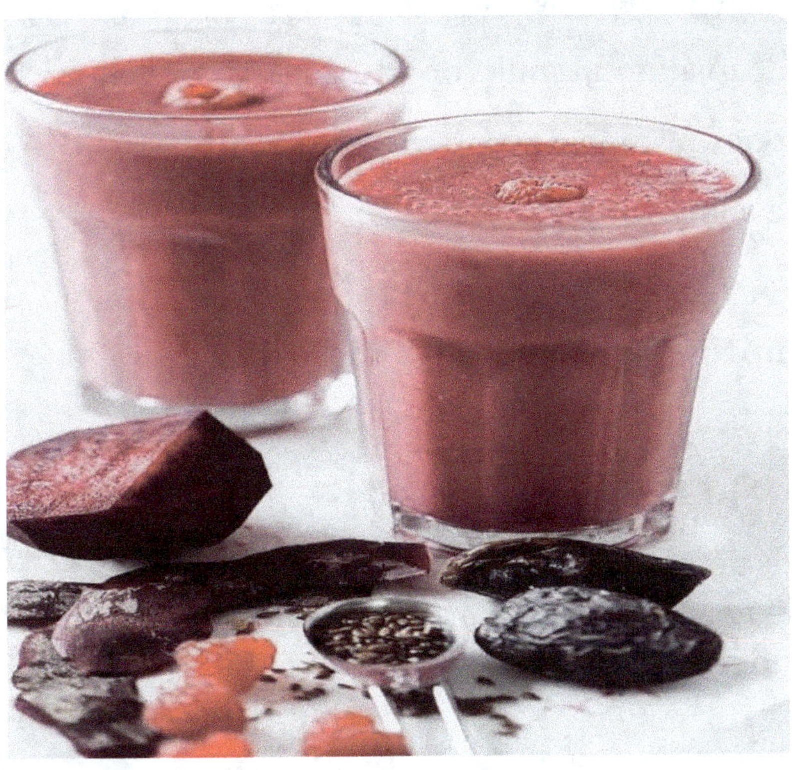

14. Apple Cinnamon Smoothie

Ingredients:

- 1 medium-sized apple, cored and chopped

- ½ teaspoon ground cinnamon

- ¼ cup rolled oats

- ½ cup Greek yogurt

- ½ cup almond milk (or any milk of your choice)

- Honey or maple syrup to taste (optional)

- Ice cubes (optional)

Minutes for Preparation: 5 minutes

How to Prepare:

1. Place the chopped apple, ground cinnamon, rolled oats, Greek yogurt, and almond milk in a blender.

2. Optionally, add honey or maple syrup for sweetness.

3. If desired, add some ice cubes for a colder smoothie.

4. Blend all the ingredients until smooth and creamy.

5. Taste the smoothie and adjust sweetness if needed by adding more honey or maple syrup.

6. Blend again until well combined.

7. Pour the smoothie into glasses and serve immediately.

Health Benefits in Ramadan:

- Fiber: Apples and oats are both high in fiber, which promotes digestive health and helps keep you feeling full and satisfied during fasting.

- Vitamins and Minerals: Apples are rich in vitamin C and various antioxidants, while oats provide essential nutrients like iron and magnesium, supporting overall health during Ramadan.

- Blood Sugar Regulation: Cinnamon may help regulate blood sugar levels, which can be beneficial during fasting periods.

- Energy Boost: The natural sugars in apples and oats provide a sustained energy release, helping to keep you energized throughout the day.

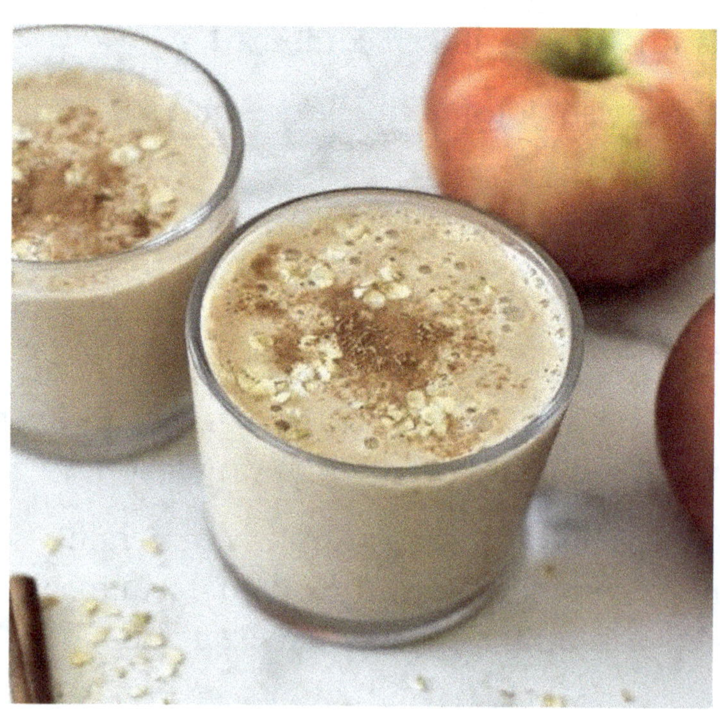

15. Strawberry Kiwi Smoothie

Ingredients:

- 1 cup strawberries, hulled and halved

- 2 ripe kiwis, peeled and chopped

- ½ banana

- ½ cup Greek yogurt

- ½ cup coconut water (or any liquid of your choice)

- Honey or maple syrup to taste (optional)

- Ice cubes (optional)

Minutes for Preparation: 5 minutes

How to Prepare:

1. Place the strawberries, chopped kiwis, banana, Greek yogurt, and coconut water in a blender.

2. Optionally, add honey or maple syrup for sweetness.

3. If desired, add some ice cubes for a colder smoothie.

4. Blend all the ingredients until smooth and creamy.

5. Taste the smoothie and adjust sweetness if needed by adding more honey or maple syrup.

6. Blend again until well combined.

7. Pour the smoothie into glasses and serve immediately.

Health Benefits in Ramadan:

- Hydration: Both strawberries and kiwis have high water content, contributing to hydration during fasting.

- Vitamins and Minerals: Strawberries are rich in vitamin C, while kiwis provide vitamin K, potassium, and fiber, offering essential nutrients during Ramadan.

- Digestive Health: Both strawberries and kiwis contain fiber, promoting digestive health and regular bowel movements, which can be beneficial during Ramadan.

- Antioxidants: Strawberries and kiwis are packed with antioxidants, which help fight inflammation and oxidative stress in the body, supporting overall health during Ramadan.

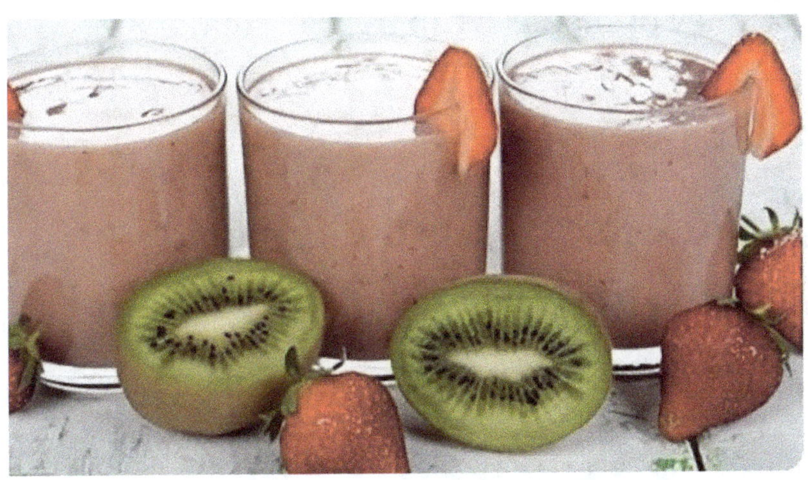

16. Peanut Butter Banana Smoothie

Ingredients:

- 1 ripe banana

- 2 tablespoons peanut butter

- ½ cup Greek yogurt

- ½ cup milk (dairy or plant-based)

- Honey or maple syrup to taste (optional)

- Ice cubes (optional)

Minutes for Preparation: 5 minutes

How to Prepare:

1. Peel the banana and break it into chunks.

2. Add the banana chunks to a blender.

3. Spoon in the peanut butter.

4. Pour in the Greek yogurt and milk.

5. Optionally, add honey or maple syrup for sweetness.

6. If desired, add some ice cubes for a colder smoothie.

7. Blend all the ingredients until smooth and creamy.

8. Taste the smoothie and adjust sweetness if needed by adding more honey or maple syrup.

9. Blend again until well combined.

10. Pour the smoothie into glasses and serve immediately.

Health Benefits in Ramadan:

- Protein and Healthy Fats: Peanut butter provides protein and healthy fats, helping to keep you feeling full and satisfied during fasting.

- Potassium: Bananas are rich in potassium, which helps maintain electrolyte balance and prevent muscle cramps during fasting.

- Digestive Health: Bananas contain fiber, promoting digestive health and regular bowel movements, which can be beneficial during Ramadan.

- Energy Boost: The natural sugars in bananas provide a quick energy boost during fasting hours.

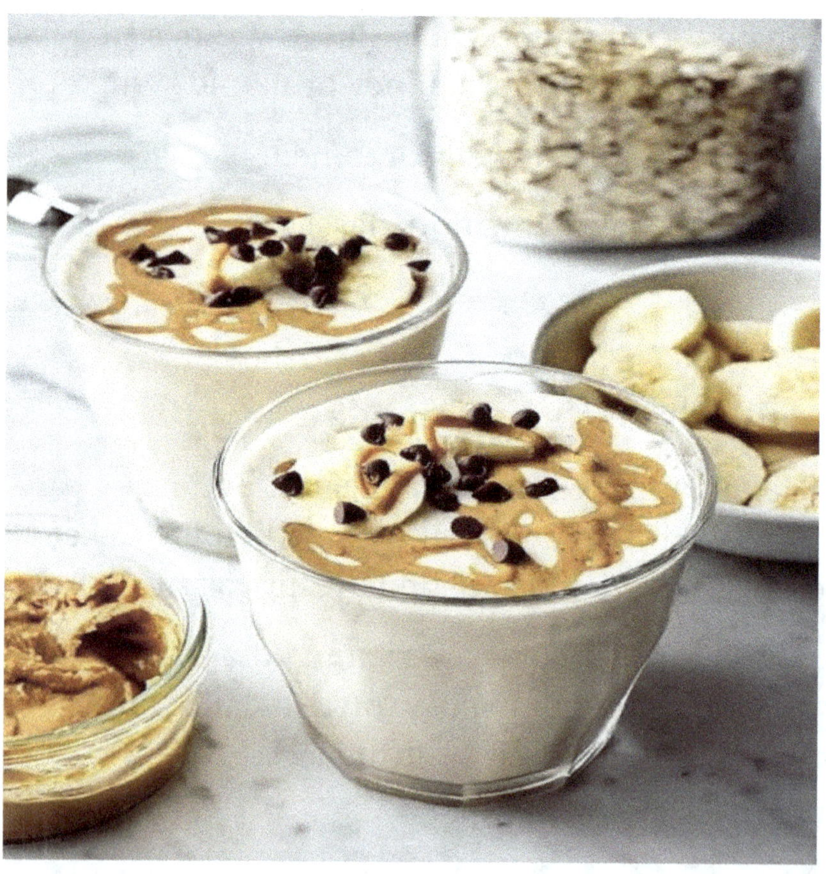

17. Mixed Berry Chia Smoothie

Ingredients:

- 1 cup mixed berries (such as strawberries, blueberries, raspberries)

- 1 tablespoon chia seeds

- ½ cup Greek yogurt

- ½ cup almond milk (or any milk of your choice)

- Honey or maple syrup to taste (optional)

- Ice cubes (optional)

Minutes for Preparation: 5 minutes

How to Prepare:

1. Place the mixed berries, chia seeds, Greek yogurt, and almond milk in a blender.

2. Optionally, add honey or maple syrup for sweetness.

3. If desired, add some ice cubes for a colder smoothie.

4. Blend all the ingredients until smooth and creamy.

5. Taste the smoothie and adjust sweetness if needed by adding more honey or maple syrup.

6. Blend again until well combined.

7. Let the smoothie sit for a few minutes to allow the chia seeds to thicken.

8. Pour the smoothie into glasses and serve immediately.

Health Benefits in Ramadan:

- Antioxidants: Mixed berries are rich in antioxidants, which help fight inflammation and oxidative stress in the body, supporting overall health during Ramadan.

- Fiber: Chia seeds are high in fiber, promoting digestive health and regular bowel movements, which can be beneficial during Ramadan.

- Protein: Greek yogurt provides protein, helping to keep you feeling full and satisfied during fasting.

- Hydration: Berries have high water content, contributing to hydration during fasting.

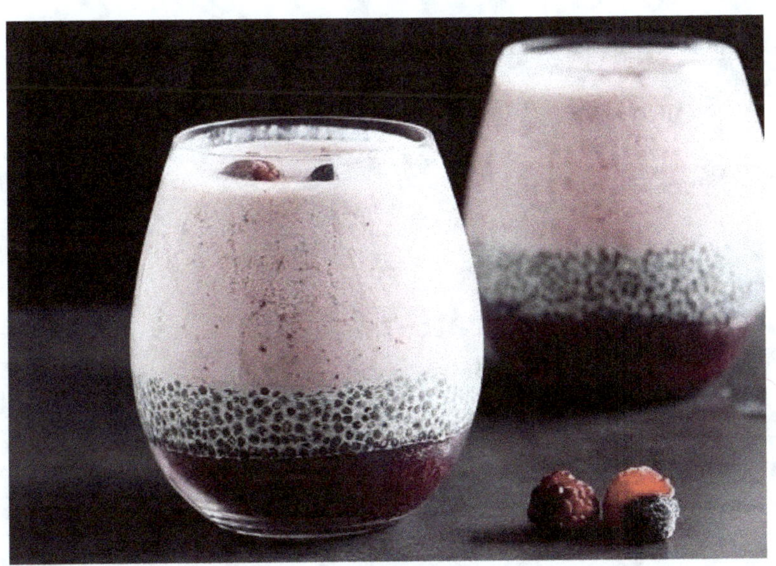

18. Chocolate Almond Smoothie

Ingredients:

- 1 tablespoon cocoa powder

- 1 tablespoon almond butter

- 1 ripe banana

- ½ cup almond milk (or any milk of your choice)

- Honey or maple syrup to taste (optional)

- Ice cubes (optional)

Minutes for Preparation: 5 minutes

How to Prepare:

1. Peel the banana and break it into chunks.

2. Place the banana chunks in a blender.

3. Add the cocoa powder and almond butter to the blender.

4. Pour in the almond milk.

5. Optionally, add honey or maple syrup for sweetness.

6. If desired, add some ice cubes for a colder smoothie.

7. Blend all the ingredients until smooth and creamy.

8. Taste the smoothie and adjust sweetness if needed by adding more honey or maple syrup.

9. Blend again until well combined.

10. Pour the smoothie into glasses and serve immediately.

Health Benefits in Ramadan:

- Protein and Healthy Fats: Almond butter provides protein and healthy fats, helping to keep you feeling full and satisfied during fasting.

- Potassium: Bananas are rich in potassium, which helps maintain electrolyte balance and prevent muscle cramps during fasting.

- Antioxidants: Cocoa powder contains antioxidants, which help fight inflammation and oxidative stress in the body, supporting overall health during Ramadan.

- Energy Boost: The natural sugars in bananas provide a quick energy boost during fasting hours.

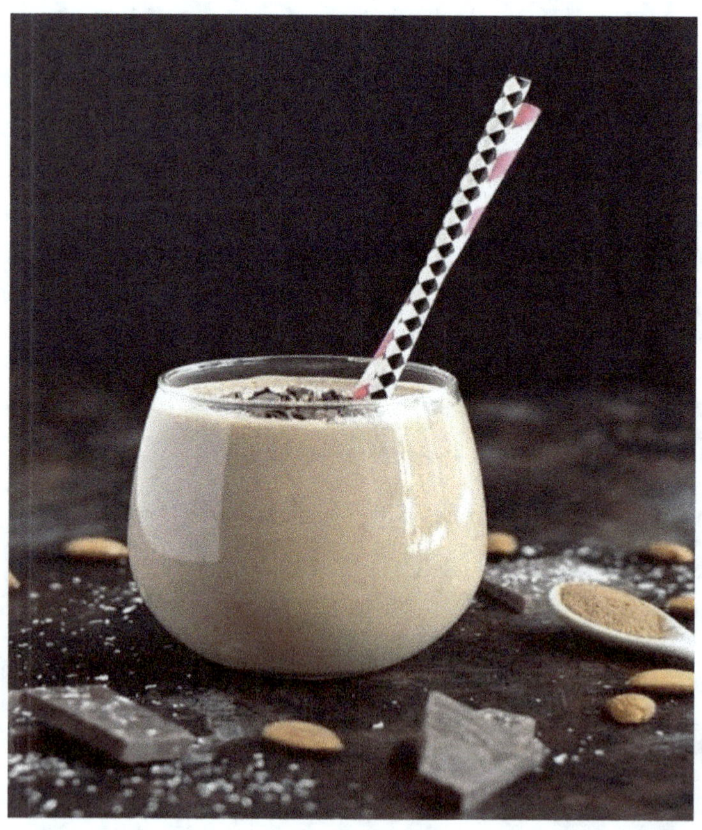

19. Tropical Green Smoothie

Ingredients:

- 1 cup fresh spinach leaves

- ½ cup chopped pineapple

- ½ cup chopped mango

- ½ banana

- ½ cup coconut water (or any liquid of your choice)

- Juice of ½ lime

- Honey or maple syrup to taste (optional)

- Ice cubes (optional)

Minutes for Preparation: 5 minutes

How to Prepare:

1. Place the spinach leaves, chopped pineapple, chopped mango, banana, coconut water, and lime juice in a blender.

2. Optionally, add honey or maple syrup for sweetness.

3. If desired, add some ice cubes for a colder smoothie.

4. Blend all the ingredients until smooth and creamy.

5. Taste the smoothie and adjust sweetness if needed by adding more honey or maple syrup.

6. Blend again until well combined.

7. Pour the smoothie into glasses and serve immediately.

Health Benefits in Ramadan:

- Hydration: Pineapple, mango, and coconut water have high water content, contributing to hydration during fasting.

- Vitamins and Minerals: Spinach is rich in vitamins A, C, and K, as well as iron and folate, while pineapple and mango provide vitamin C and other essential nutrients, supporting overall health during Ramadan.

- Digestive Health: Spinach and pineapple contain fiber, promoting digestive health and regular bowel movements, which can be beneficial during Ramadan.

- Antioxidants: Mangoes and pineapples are packed with antioxidants, which help fight inflammation and oxidative stress in the body, supporting overall health during Ramadan.

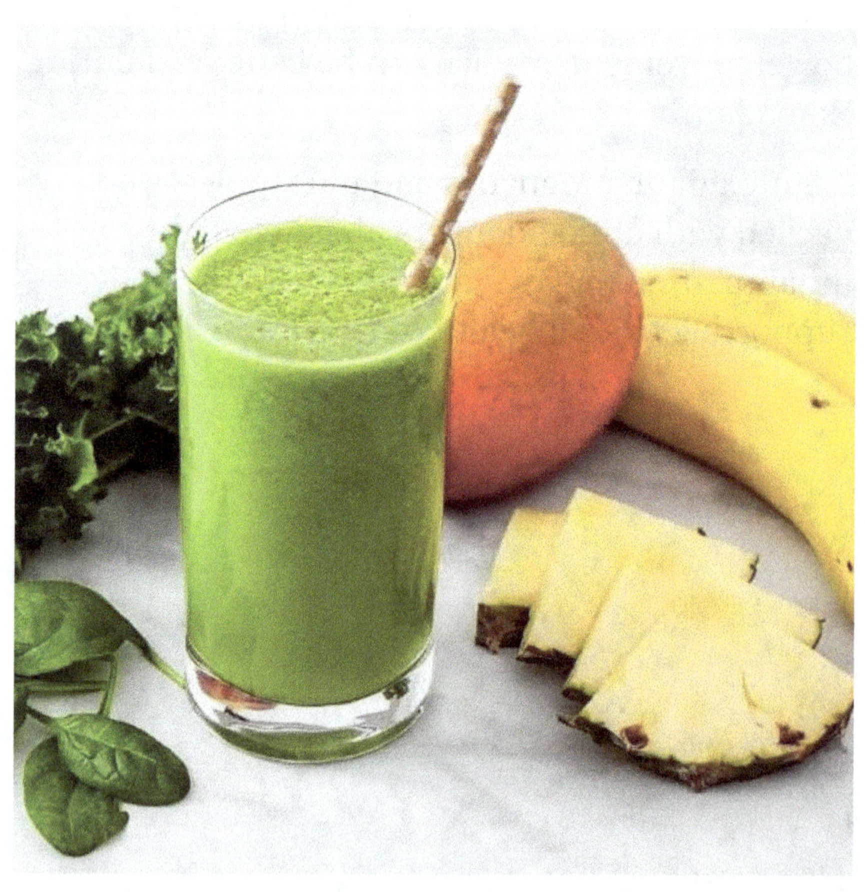

20. Matcha Green Tea Smoothie

Ingredients:

- 1 teaspoon matcha powder

- 1 banana

- ½ cup Greek yogurt

- ½ cup almond milk (or any milk of your choice)

- Honey or maple syrup to taste (optional)

- Ice cubes (optional)

Minutes for Preparation: 5 minutes

How to Prepare:

1. Peel the banana and break it into chunks.

2. Place the banana chunks in a blender.

3. Add the matcha powder, Greek yogurt, and almond milk to the blender.

4. Optionally, add honey or maple syrup for sweetness.

5. If desired, add some ice cubes for a colder smoothie.

6. Blend all the ingredients until smooth and creamy.

7. Taste the smoothie and adjust sweetness if needed by adding more honey or maple syrup.

8. Blend again until well combined.

9. Pour the smoothie into glasses and serve immediately.

Health Benefits in Ramadan:

- Antioxidants: Matcha powder is rich in antioxidants, which help fight inflammation and oxidative stress in the body, supporting overall health during Ramadan.

- Energy Boost: Matcha contains caffeine, providing a natural energy boost during fasting hours.

- Digestive Health: Bananas are high in fiber, promoting digestive health and regular bowel movements, which can be beneficial during Ramadan.

- Hydration: Almond milk has high water content, contributing to hydration during fasting.

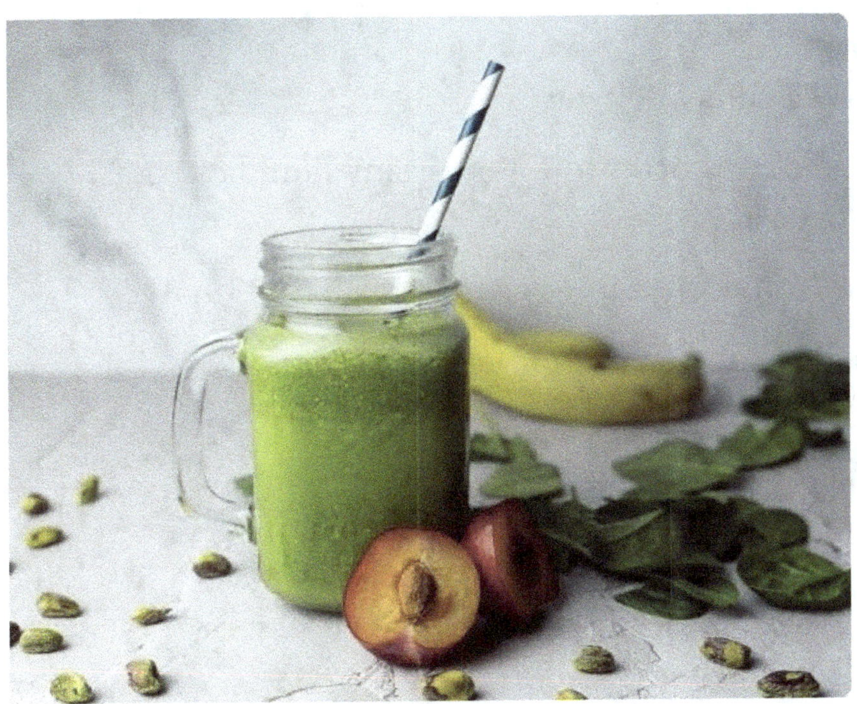

21. Pomegranate Berry Smoothie

Ingredients:

- ½ cup pomegranate seeds

- ½ cup mixed berries (such as strawberries, blueberries, raspberries)

- ½ banana

- ½ cup Greek yogurt

- ½ cup coconut water (or any liquid of your choice)

- Honey or maple syrup to taste (optional)

- Ice cubes (optional)

Minutes for Preparation: 5 minutes

How to Prepare:

1. Place the pomegranate seeds, mixed berries, banana, Greek yogurt, and coconut water in a blender.

2. Optionally, add honey or maple syrup for sweetness.

3. If desired, add some ice cubes for a colder smoothie.

4. Blend all the ingredients until smooth and creamy.

5. Taste the smoothie and adjust sweetness if needed by adding more honey or maple syrup.

6. Blend again until well combined.

7. Pour the smoothie into glasses and serve immediately.

Health Benefits in Ramadan:

- Antioxidants: Pomegranate seeds and mixed berries are rich in antioxidants, which help fight inflammation and oxidative stress in the body, supporting overall health during Ramadan.

- Vitamins and Minerals: Berries are packed with vitamin C and other essential nutrients, while pomegranate seeds provide vitamins A, C, and E, supporting overall health during Ramadan.

- Digestive Health: Berries are high in fiber, promoting digestive health and regular bowel movements, which can be beneficial during Ramadan.

- Hydration: Coconut water has high water content, contributing to hydration during fasting.

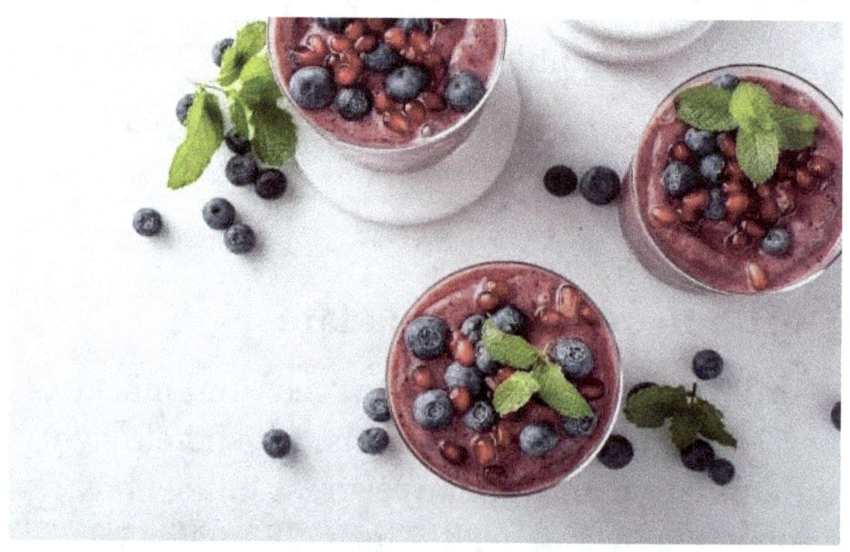

22. Vanilla Almond Smoothie

Ingredients:

- ½ teaspoon vanilla extract

- 1 tablespoon almond butter

- 1 ripe banana

- ½ cup Greek yogurt

- ½ cup almond milk (or any milk of your choice)

- Honey or maple syrup to taste (optional)

- Ice cubes (optional)

Minutes for Preparation: 5 minutes

How to Prepare:

1. Peel the banana and break it into chunks.

2. Place the banana chunks in a blender.

3. Add the vanilla extract, almond butter, Greek yogurt, and almond milk to the blender.

4. Optionally, add honey or maple syrup for sweetness.

5. If desired, add some ice cubes for a colder smoothie.

6. Blend all the ingredients until smooth and creamy.

7. Taste the smoothie and adjust sweetness if needed by adding more honey or maple syrup.

8. Blend again until well combined.

9. Pour the smoothie into glasses and serve immediately.

Health Benefits in Ramadan:

- Protein and Healthy Fats: Almond butter provides protein and healthy fats, helping to keep you feeling full and satisfied during fasting.

- Potassium: Bananas are rich in potassium, which helps maintain electrolyte balance and prevent muscle cramps during fasting.

- Digestive Health: Bananas contain fiber, promoting digestive health and regular bowel movements, which can be beneficial during Ramadan.

- Energy Boost: The natural sugars in bananas provide a quick energy boost during fasting hours.

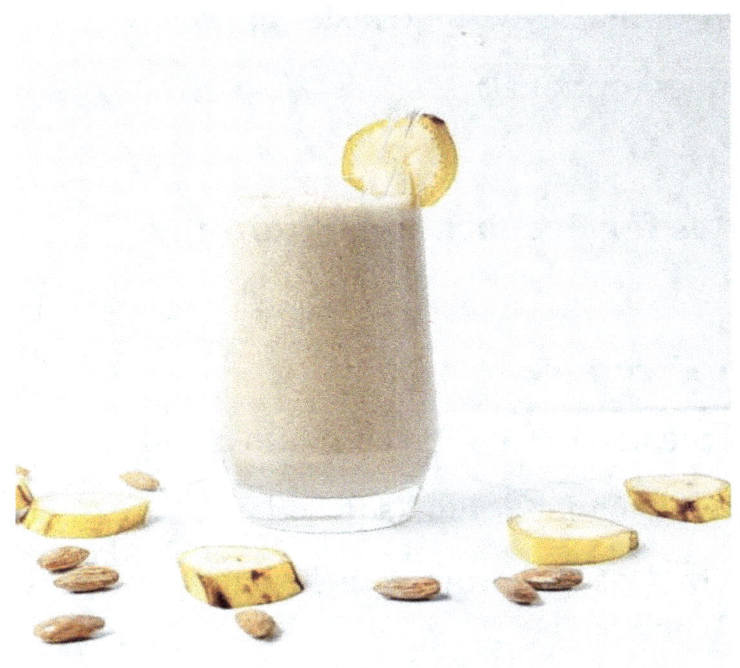

23. Chocolate Banana Smoothie

Ingredients:

- 1 ripe banana

- 1 tablespoon cocoa powder

- ½ cup Greek yogurt

- ½ cup milk (dairy or plant-based)

- Honey or maple syrup to taste (optional)

- Ice cubes (optional)

Minutes for Preparation: 5 minutes

How to Prepare:

1. Peel the banana and break it into chunks.

2. Place the banana chunks in a blender.

3. Add the cocoa powder, Greek yogurt, and milk to the blender.

4. Optionally, add honey or maple syrup for sweetness.

5. If desired, add some ice cubes for a colder smoothie.

6. Blend all the ingredients until smooth and creamy.

7. Taste the smoothie and adjust sweetness if needed by adding more honey or maple syrup.

8. Blend again until well combined.

9. Pour the smoothie into glasses and serve immediately.

Health Benefits in Ramadan:

- Protein and Calcium: Greek yogurt provides protein and calcium, helping to keep you feeling full and supporting bone health during fasting.

- Potassium: Bananas are rich in potassium, which helps maintain electrolyte balance and prevent muscle cramps during fasting.

- Antioxidants: Cocoa powder contains antioxidants, which help fight inflammation and oxidative stress in the body, supporting overall health during Ramadan.

- Energy Boost: The natural sugars in bananas provide a quick energy boost during fasting hours.

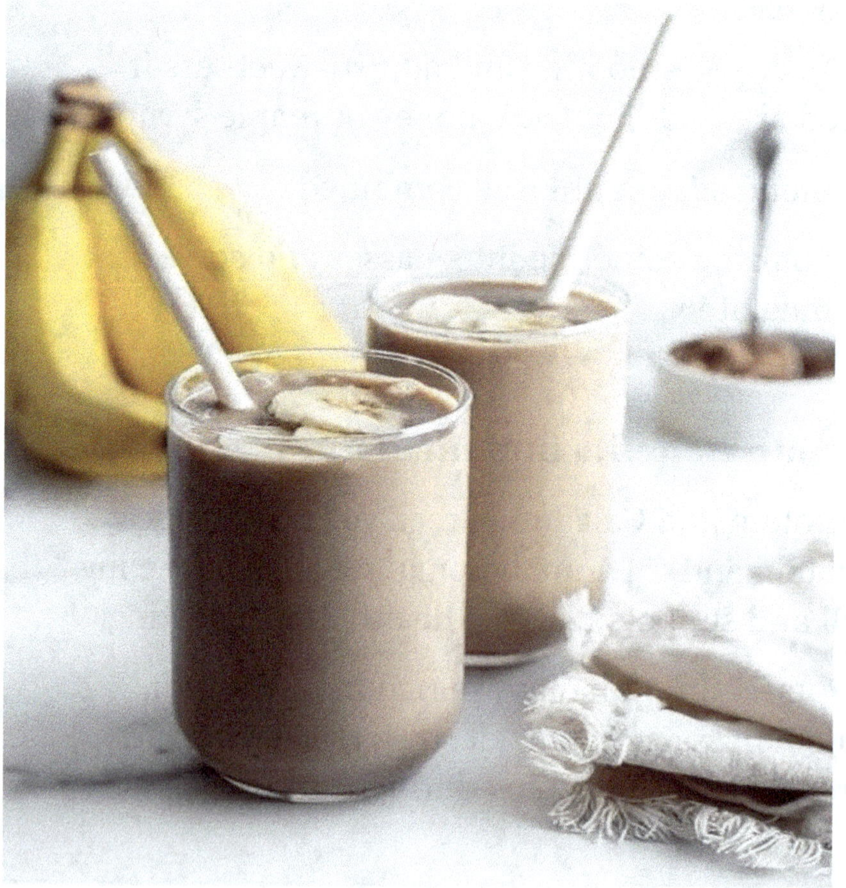

24. Cantaloupe Mint Smoothie

Ingredients:

- 1 cup chopped cantaloupe

- Handful of fresh mint leaves

- ½ cup Greek yogurt

- ½ cup coconut water (or any liquid of your choice)

- Honey or maple syrup to taste (optional)

- Ice cubes (optional)

Minutes for Preparation: 5 minutes

How to Prepare:

1. Place the chopped cantaloupe, fresh mint leaves, Greek yogurt, and coconut water in a blender.

2. Optionally, add honey or maple syrup for sweetness.

3. If desired, add some ice cubes for a colder smoothie.

4. Blend all the ingredients until smooth and creamy.

5. Taste the smoothie and adjust sweetness if needed by adding more honey or maple syrup.

6. Blend again until well combined.

7. Pour the smoothie into glasses and serve immediately.

Health Benefits in Ramadan:

- Hydration: Cantaloupe and coconut water have high water content, contributing to hydration during fasting.

- Vitamins and Minerals: Cantaloupe is rich in vitamin A, vitamin C, and potassium, while mint provides vitamins and minerals like vitamin A and iron, supporting overall health during Ramadan.

- Digestive Health: Mint helps soothe the stomach and aids digestion, which can be beneficial during Ramadan, especially after breaking the fast.

- Refreshing: The combination of cantaloupe and mint provides a refreshing flavor, helping to combat thirst and refresh the palate during fasting hours.

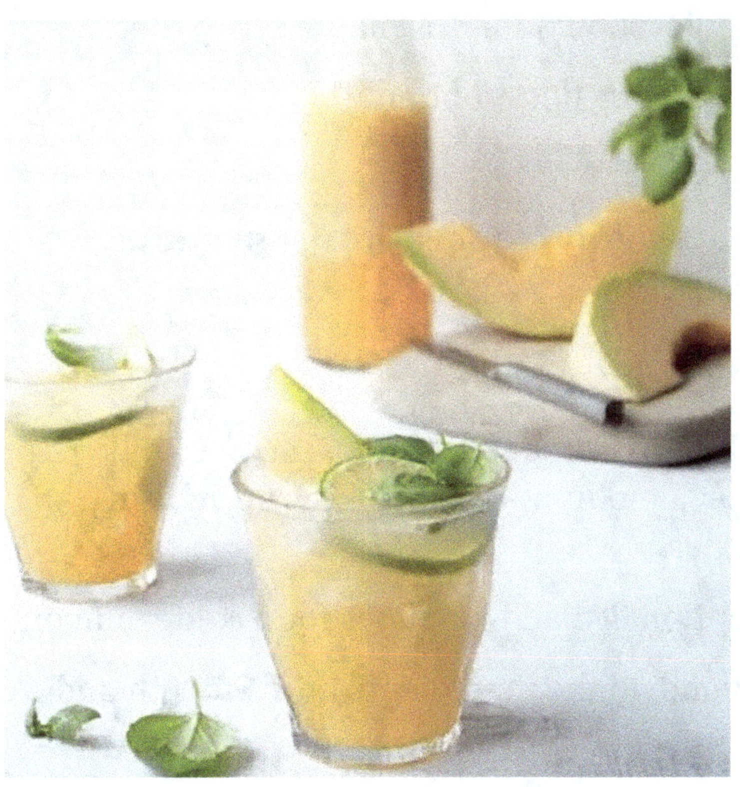

25. Coconut Mango Smoothie

Ingredients:

- 1 ripe mango, peeled and chopped

- ½ cup coconut milk

- ½ cup Greek yogurt

- 1 tablespoon honey or maple syrup (optional)

- ½ cup ice cubes (optional)

Minutes for Preparation: 5 minutes

How to Prepare:

1. Place the chopped mango, coconut milk, Greek yogurt, and honey or maple syrup (if using) in a blender.

2. Optionally, add ice cubes for a colder smoothie.

3. Blend all the ingredients until smooth and creamy.

4. Taste the smoothie and adjust sweetness if needed by adding more honey or maple syrup.

5. Blend again until well combined.

6. Pour the smoothie into glasses and serve immediately.

Health Benefits in Ramadan:

- Hydration: Mangoes and coconut milk have high water content, contributing to hydration during fasting.

- Vitamins and Minerals: Mangoes are rich in vitamins A and C, while coconut milk provides essential nutrients like potassium and magnesium, supporting overall health during Ramadan.

- Digestive Health: Coconut milk contains medium-chain triglycerides (MCTs) which may aid in digestion and promote gut health, beneficial during Ramadan.

- Energy Boost: The natural sugars in mangoes provide a quick energy boost during fasting hours.

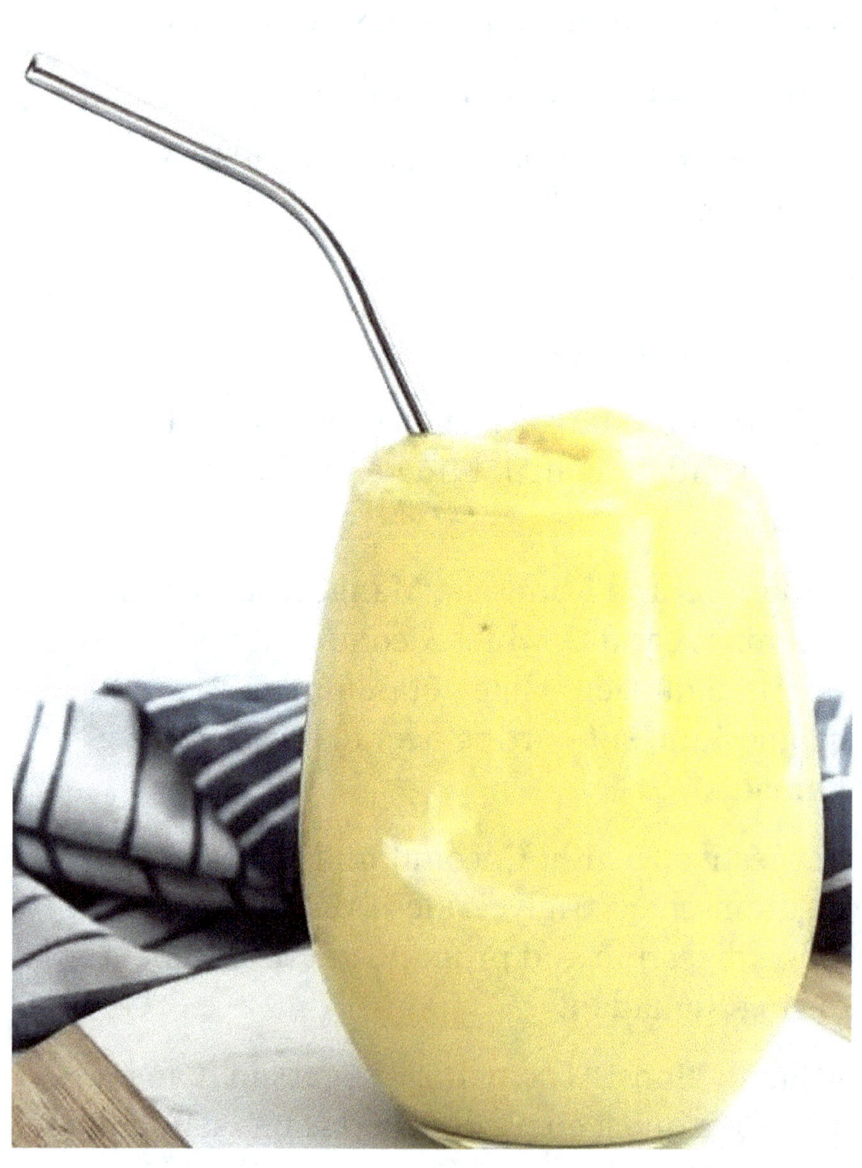

26. Grapefruit Ginger Smoothie

Ingredients:

- 1 grapefruit, peeled and segmented

- 1 teaspoon grated ginger

- ½ banana

- ½ cup Greek yogurt

- ½ cup coconut water (or any liquid of your choice)

- Honey or maple syrup to taste (optional)

- Ice cubes (optional)

Minutes for Preparation: 5 minutes

How to Prepare:

1. Place the grapefruit segments, grated ginger, banana, Greek yogurt, and coconut water in a blender.

2. Optionally, add honey or maple syrup for sweetness.

3. If desired, add some ice cubes for a colder smoothie.

4. Blend all the ingredients until smooth and creamy.

5. Taste the smoothie and adjust sweetness if needed by adding more honey or maple syrup.

6. Blend again until well combined.

7. Pour the smoothie into glasses and serve immediately.

Health Benefits in Ramadan:

- Hydration: Grapefruit and coconut water have high water content, contributing to hydration during fasting.

- Vitamin C: Grapefruit is rich in vitamin C, which supports the immune system, helping to prevent illness during Ramadan.

- Digestive Health: Ginger helps soothe the stomach and aids digestion, which can be beneficial during Ramadan, especially after breaking the fast.

- Refreshing: The combination of grapefruit and ginger provides a refreshing flavor, helping to combat thirst and refresh the palate during fasting hours.

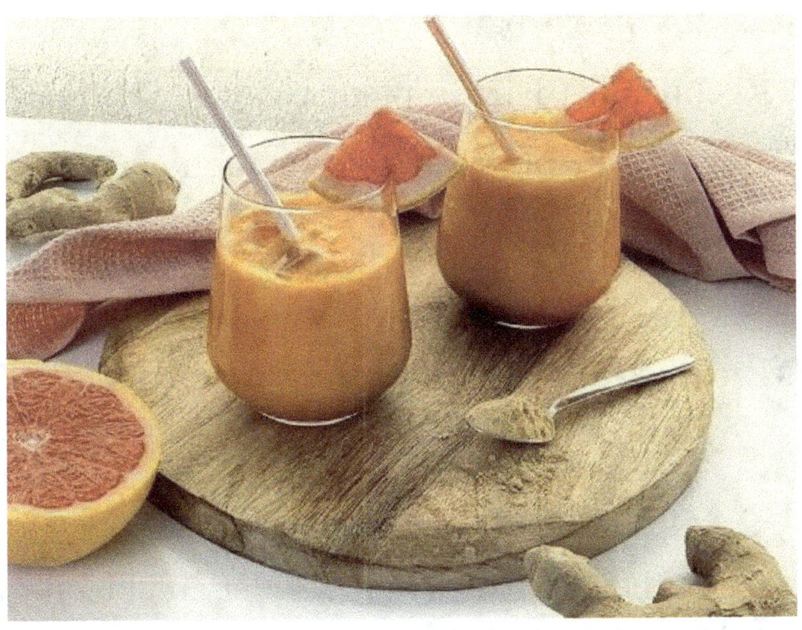

27. Oatmeal Cookie Smoothie

Ingredients:

- ½ cup rolled oats

- 1 ripe banana

- 1 tablespoon almond butter

- ½ teaspoon ground cinnamon

- ½ cup Greek yogurt

- ½ cup milk (dairy or plant-based)

- Honey or maple syrup to taste (optional)

- Ice cubes (optional)

Minutes for Preparation: 5 minutes

How to Prepare:

1. Place the rolled oats in a blender and blend until finely ground.

2. Add the ripe banana, almond butter, ground cinnamon, Greek yogurt, and milk to the blender.

3. Optionally, add honey or maple syrup for sweetness.

4. If desired, add some ice cubes for a colder smoothie.

5. Blend all the ingredients until smooth and creamy.

6. Taste the smoothie and adjust sweetness if needed by adding more honey or maple syrup.

7. Blend again until well combined.

8. Pour the smoothie into glasses and serve immediately.

Health Benefits in Ramadan:

- Protein and Healthy Fats: Almond butter provides protein and healthy fats, helping to keep you feeling full and satisfied during fasting.

- Carbohydrates: Rolled oats provide complex carbohydrates, providing sustained energy release during fasting hours.

- Digestive Health: Rolled oats are high in fiber, promoting digestive health and regular bowel movements, which can be beneficial during Ramadan.

- Vitamins and Minerals: Bananas are rich in potassium, while Greek yogurt provides calcium and probiotics, supporting overall health during Ramadan.

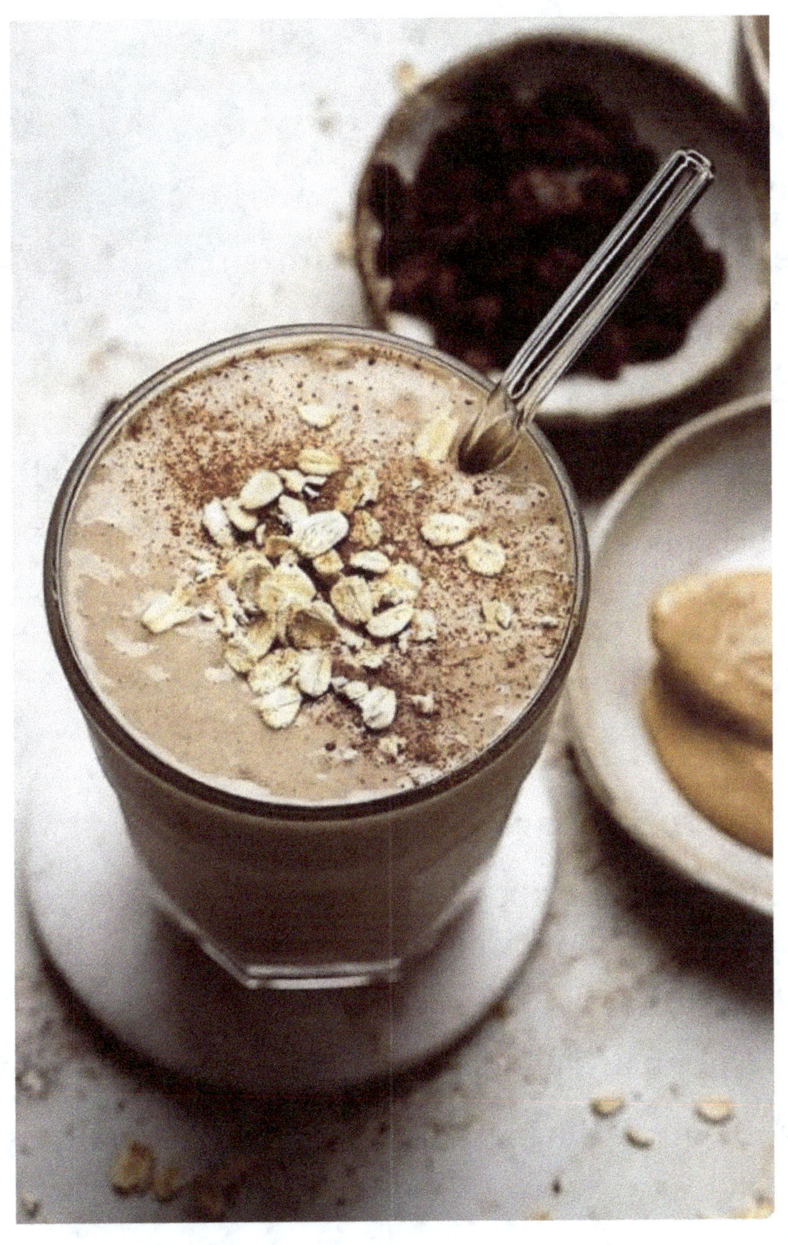

28. Raspberry Coconut Smoothie

Ingredients:

- 1 cup raspberries (fresh or frozen)

- ½ cup coconut milk

- ½ cup Greek yogurt

- 1 tablespoon honey or maple syrup (optional)

- Ice cubes (optional)

Minutes for Preparation: 5 minutes

How to Prepare:

1. Place the raspberries, coconut milk, Greek yogurt, and honey or maple syrup (if using) in a blender.

2. Optionally, add ice cubes for a colder smoothie.

3. Blend all the ingredients until smooth and creamy.

4. Taste the smoothie and adjust sweetness if needed by adding more honey or maple syrup.

5. Blend again until well combined.

6. Pour the smoothie into glasses and serve immediately.

Health Benefits in Ramadan:

- Hydration: Raspberries and coconut milk have high water content, contributing to hydration during fasting.

- Vitamins and Minerals: Raspberries are rich in vitamin C and manganese, while coconut milk provides essential nutrients like iron and copper, supporting overall health during Ramadan.

- Digestive Health: Raspberries contain fiber, promoting digestive health and regular bowel movements, which can be beneficial during Ramadan.

- Antioxidants: Raspberries are packed with antioxidants, which help fight inflammation and oxidative stress in the body, supporting overall health during Ramadan.

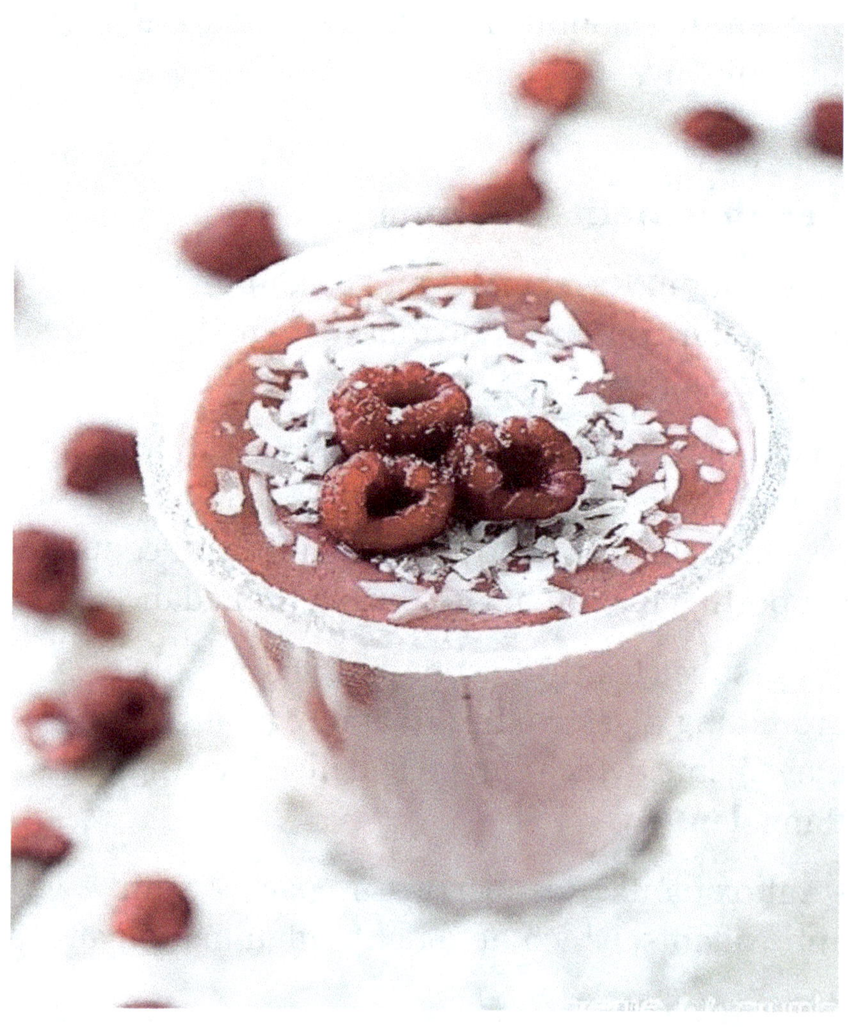

29. Turmeric Mango Smoothie

Ingredients:

- 1 ripe mango, peeled and diced

- ½ teaspoon ground turmeric

- ½ cup Greek yogurt

- ½ cup almond milk (or any milk of your choice)

- 1 tablespoon honey or maple syrup (optional)

- Ice cubes (optional)

Minutes for Preparation: 5 minutes

How to Prepare:

1. Place the diced mango, ground turmeric, Greek yogurt, almond milk, and honey or maple syrup (if using) in a blender.

2. Optionally, add ice cubes for a colder smoothie.

3. Blend all the ingredients until smooth and creamy.

4. Taste the smoothie and adjust sweetness if needed by adding more honey or maple syrup.

5. Blend again until well combined.

6. Pour the smoothie into glasses and serve immediately.

Health Benefits in Ramadan:

- Vitamins and Minerals: Mangoes are rich in vitamins A and C, while turmeric provides antioxidants and has anti-inflammatory properties, supporting overall health during Ramadan.

- Digestive Health: Turmeric aids digestion and may help alleviate digestive discomfort during fasting hours.

- Hydration: Mangoes and almond milk have high water content, contributing to hydration during fasting.

- Protein: Greek yogurt provides protein, helping to keep you feeling full and satisfied during fasting.

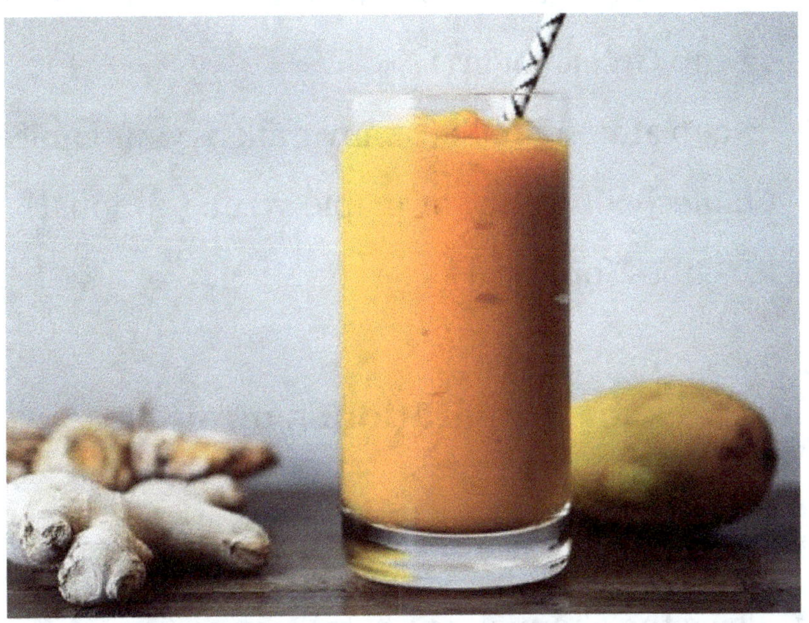

30. Apricot Cardamom Smoothie

Ingredients:

- 1 cup chopped apricots (fresh or dried)

- ½ teaspoon ground cardamom

- ½ cup Greek yogurt

- ½ cup almond milk (or any milk of your choice)

- 1 tablespoon honey or maple syrup (optional)

- Ice cubes (optional)

Minutes for Preparation: 5 minutes

How to Prepare:

1. Place the chopped apricots, ground cardamom, Greek yogurt, almond milk, and honey or maple syrup (if using) in a blender.

2. Optionally, add ice cubes for a colder smoothie.

3. Blend all the ingredients until smooth and creamy.

4. Taste the smoothie and adjust sweetness if needed by adding more honey or maple syrup.

5. Blend again until well combined.

6. Pour the smoothie into glasses and serve immediately.

Health Benefits in Ramadan:

- Vitamins and Minerals: Apricots are rich in vitamins A and C, potassium, and fiber, while cardamom provides antioxidants and aids digestion, supporting overall health during Ramadan.

- Digestive Health: Cardamom is known for its digestive properties and can help alleviate digestive discomfort during fasting hours.

- Hydration: Apricots and almond milk have high water content, contributing to hydration during fasting.

- Protein: Greek yogurt provides protein, helping to keep you feeling full and satisfied during fasting.

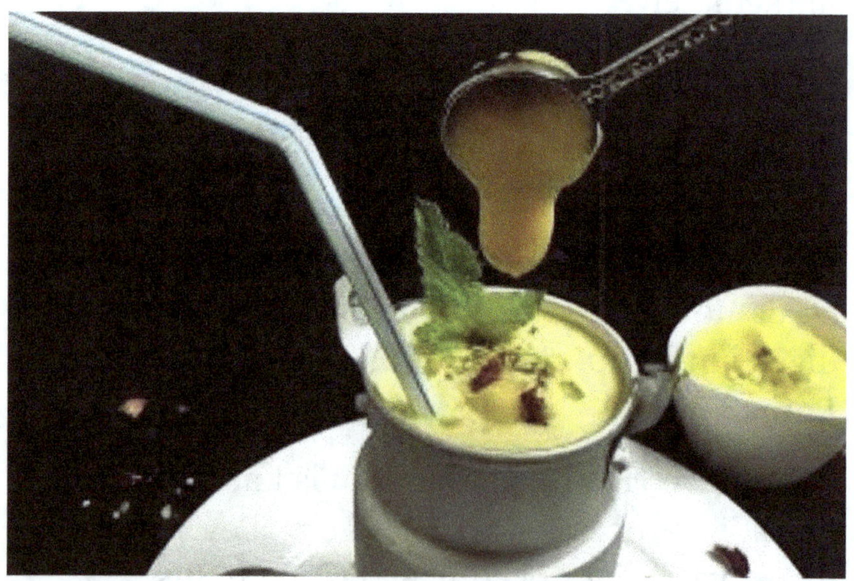

Conclusion

As our journey through Ramadan comes to a close, we hope that "30 Easy Smoothie Recipes for Ramadan" has provided you with inspiration and guidance to support your fasting experience. Breaking fasts with nutritious and delicious smoothies can not only replenish your energy levels but also nourish your body with essential nutrients, vitamins, and hydration.

Throughout this book, we've explored a variety of flavor combinations and ingredients that cater to different tastes and dietary preferences. Whether you've enjoyed the refreshing taste of tropical fruits, the comforting warmth of spices, or the creaminess of nut butters, each smoothie recipe has been crafted with care to enhance your Ramadan fasts.

As you continue on your journey of spiritual reflection and self-discipline, remember that nourishing your body is an integral part of the fasting experience. By incorporating nutrient-rich smoothies into your diet, you can support your overall health and well-being while honoring the traditions of Ramadan.

We encourage you to experiment with these recipes, customize them to your liking, and share them with your loved ones. May these smoothies continue to be a source of joy, vitality, and sustenance for you during Ramadan and beyond.

Wishing you a blessed Ramadan filled with peace, prosperity, and abundant blessings.

Ramadan Mubarak!